"By bringing together learning from extensive professional experience, first-person insights, and current research, Working with AAC provides a comprehensive resource for busy clinicians. This book offers an innovative and accessible framework that will support and enhance the practice of anyone who works with people who use, or who could benefit from using, AAC."

– **Dr Katherine Broomfield**, *Cardiff Metropolitan University and North Bristol NHS Trust*

"This text is a welcome and timely addition to the AAC literature. It will support students in their learning and clinicians in their practice."

– **Janice Murray**, *Professor Emeritus, Manchester Metropolitan University, UK*

Access your Online Resources

Working with AAC is accompanied by a number of printable online materials, designed to ensure this resource best supports your professional needs

Go to https://resourcecentre.routledge.com/speechmark and click on the cover of this book

Answer the question prompt using your copy of the book to gain access to the online content.

Working with AAC

This book demystifies the world of Augmentative and Alternative Communication (AAC) in speech and language therapy, explaining key terminology and guiding clinicians through the research underpinning successful clinical practice. Spanning a range of clinical groups and all ages, it introduces a holistic framework to support clinicians along the journey from assessment to implementation. Key features include:

- Current research and evidence-based practice broken down into accessible chunks.
- Clear, easy to read explanations of the components of AAC systems and their importance.
- An insight into the challenges faced when supporting AAC users and solutions to overcome these.
- The voices of aided communicators woven throughout, re-telling their experiences and how clinicians can best support them to use AAC.
- Photocopiable clinical resources, including assessment checklists and advice sheets for families and people who use AAC.

Rooted in lived experience, this book suggests practical solutions for supporting a person to have a positive experience of being an aided communicator. It is an invaluable resource for experienced clinicians, speech and language therapists and allied professionals, as well as those new to the world of AAC both now and in years to come.

Helen Robinson is a Speech and Language Therapist and AAC Service Lead for the Barnsley Assistive Technology Team, delivering specialised AAC services for Yorkshire and Humberside. She has presented on AAC at international conferences and written numerous articles for the Communication Matters journal.

The *Working With* Series

The *Working With* series provides speech and language therapists with a range of 'go-to' resources, full of well-sourced, up-to-date information regarding specific disorders. Underpinned by robust theoretical foundations and supported by intervention options and exercises, every book ensures that the reader has access to the latest thinking regarding diagnosis, management and treatment options.

Written in a fully accessible style, each book bridges theory and practice and offers ready-to-use and well-rehearsed practical material, including guidance on interventions, management advice, and therapeutic resources for the client, parent or carer. The series is an invaluable resource for practitioners, whether speech and language therapy students, or more experienced clinicians.

Books in the series include:

Working with Child and Adolescent Mental Health
Susan McCool
2024 / pb: 9781032192833

Working with Adults with Eating, Drinking and Swallowing Needs
Sophie MacKenzie
2024 / pb: 9781032311982

Working with Deaf Children and Young People
Sarah Beazley and Judy Halden
2025 / pb: 9781032289311

Working with Children and Young People who Stammer, 3rd edition
Isabel O'Leary
2025 / pb: 9781032112329

Working with AAC
Helen Robinson
2026 / pb: 9781032534893

Working with ACC

A Guide for Supporting Augmentative and Alternative Communication Users

Helen Robinson

Routledge
Taylor & Francis Group
LONDON AND NEW YORK

Designed cover image: Getty Images

First published 2026
by Routledge
4 Park Square, Milton Park, Abingdon, Oxon OX14 4RN

and by Routledge
605 Third Avenue, New York, NY 10158

Routledge is an imprint of the Taylor & Francis Group, an informa business

British Library Cataloguing-in-Publication Data
A catalogue record for this book is available from the British Library

ISBN: 9781032534916 (hbk)
ISBN: 9781032534893 (pbk)
ISBN: 9781003412311 (ebk)

DOI: 10.4324/9781003412311

Typeset in Interstate
by Deanta Global Publishing Services, Chennai, India

Access the Support Material: https://resourcecentre.routledge.com/speechmark

For Shelagh Crossley and Fee Wheatcroft, who, along with four young AAC users, sparked my enthusiasm for AAC two decades ago with a game of pirate ships and have kept cheering for me ever since.

Contents

List of Tables

List of Figures

Contributors

Andrea Lee is a Speech and Language Therapist and AAC Service Lead at the Barnsley Assistive Technology Team, UK.

Joseph Doran is an AAC Consultant and Teacher working for the Ace Centre.

Ace Centre is a registered charity (No. 1089313) providing Assistive Technology Services and Augmentative and Alternative Communication services for people with complex needs. https://acecentre.org.uk

Simon Snell is an AAC user who uses a voice output communication aid with eye gaze control.

Preface

This book has pulled together my experiences working with AAC users over the past two decades. As a speech and language therapist supporting AAC users of all ages with a wide range of diagnoses and speech and language difficulties and differences, I have often felt daunted and lacked confidence in knowing how to best help them. Throughout my career I have been fortunate to be supported by some wonderful colleagues who have passed on their skills and knowledge.

During the early stages of my career, colleagues were the main source of my information. I learned how they did things and followed. There was limited information online and access to academic journals was not available to me. In more recent years I have been fortunate to develop my skills as a researcher and with that I have been able to access academic journals and books which have broadened my knowledge and complemented my clinical experience.

Nowadays, there is an overwhelming supply of information available thanks to the internet and social media. Although this is largely positive, it brings with it several issues of concern. Information can spread rapidly and influence clinical practice and keeping up with the speed at which new information is released and changes in practice can be a tricky task. It's easy for those of us working with AAC to feel lost within the sea of information. It's worth noting that my use of terminology has altered several times within the writing process and, as such, may once again become outdated after publication.

In this book, my aim has been to provide a comprehensive and understandable summary of AAC. I have hopefully given a fair and helpful overview of the key issues facing those who work with AAC users that will enable practitioners to feel confident in supporting people.

This book recognises the importance of a range of information sources; academic journals, books, professional journals and magazines, clinical experience and most importantly, lived experience. I hope that readers will feel confident to support AAC users and experience the same joy that I have in working with AAC users over the past 20 years.

Acknowledgements

This book is dedicated to all the AAC users I have had the fortune to work with over the past 20 years, who have encouraged me to learn more and do better.

Thanks also go to all my fantastic colleagues I have had the pleasure to work alongside within the Bradford Speech and Language Therapy Team, the Doncaster and Bassetlaw Speech and Language Therapy Team and the Barnsley Assistive Technology Team. Thanks also to all the education staff who have allowed me into their classrooms and responded so kindly to my ideas and suggestions.

Thank you in particular to Andrea Lee and Zoe Clarke, who have provided ongoing encouragement and enthusiasm during the writing of this book.

Thank you to Claire Robinson, not only for her support with all IT matters and the creation and formatting of the images within this book, but for the support and acceptance of me dedicating many evenings and weekends to writing this book over the past two and a half years.

I would like to thank the following people whose responses to my questionnaires and interviews have been included in this book:

Liz Allen - parent of an AAC user

Jill Clark - AAC user

Alison Felton - Speech and Language Therapist

Lindsay Hall - parent of an AAC user

Jo Holmes - former Speech and Language Therapist and parent of an AAC user

Isabelle Jones - AAC user

Andrew Mayers - AAC user

Fiona O'Driscoll - Speech and Language Therapist

Lisa Palframan - parent of an AAC user

Emily Singleton - Speech and Language Therapist

Carla Thompson - Teaching Assistant

Additional thanks go to all the other AAC users, practitioners, parents and family members who responded to my calls for support and so diligently completed my questionnaires. The insights gained from reading your valued responses have been a significant influence when writing this book.

Special thanks go to Professor Janice Murray for reviewing chapter two and for being a much-valued guide to me over the past few years.

Acronyms and abbreviations

AAC	Augmentative and Alternative Communication
ALS	Amyotrophic lateral sclerosis
ASHA	American Speech-Language-Hearing Association (ASHA)
BSL	British Sign Language
CARLA	Computer Based Accessible Receptive Language Assessment
CAS	Childhood Apraxia of Speech
CBD	Corticobasal Degeneration
CECOPS	Community Equipment Code of Practice Scheme
CP	Cerebral Palsy
DVD	Developmental Verbal Dyspraxia
EC	Environmental Controls
EDB	Equity, Diversity and Belonging
EMG	Electromyography
E-Tran	Eye Transfer Frame
GBS	Guillain-Barré syndrome
HAAT	Human Activity Assistive Technology Model
HPM	Human Performance Model
I-ASC	Identifying Appropriate Symbol Communication
IPAACS	Informing and Profiling Augmentative and Alternative Communication (AAC) Knowledge and Skills
MND	Motor Neurone Disease
MNDA	Motor Neurone Disease Association
MPT	Matching Person to Technology
MS	Multiple Sclerosis
MSA	Multiple System Atrophy
MSA-C	MSA-predominant Cerebellar Ataxia
MSA-P	MSA-predominant Parkinsonism
NHS	National Health Service

OT	Occupational Therapist
PBP	Progressive Bulbar Palsy
PECS	Picture Exchange Communication System
PLS	Primary Lateral Sclerosis
PMA	Progressive Muscular Atrophy
PMLD	Profound and Multiple Learning Disability
PODD©	Pragmatic Organisation Dynamic Display
PPA	Primary Progressive Aphasia
PROMS	Patient Reported Outcome Measures
PSP	Progressive Supranuclear Palsy
PSPA	Progressive Supranuclear Palsy Association
RCSLT	Royal College of Speech and Language Therapists
SLCN	Speech, Language and Communication Needs
SLT	Speech and Language Therapist
SM	Situational or selective mutism
SNUG	Spontaneous Novel Utterance Generation
TASP	Test of Aided Communication
TaSSeLs	Tactile Signing for Sensory Learners
UCS	User Centred Design
VOCA	Voice Output Communication Aid
VIVOCA	Voice Input Voice Output Communication Aid
VSD	Visual Scene Display

PART I

AAC users and the services they access

What is AAC and who uses it?
How do we choose which type of AAC to use?
What makes a good AAC service?

Part I considers some definitions and terminology used within the world of AAC, and how these might be both helpful and problematic. It considers who might benefit from using AAC and when might be the right time to introduce it.

Ways of understanding a person's AAC needs and models of decision-making are considered, along with how we might know when we've found the right type of AAC.

Finally, the services that support AAC users are explored, with a proposed care pathways model being outlined along with useful resources for reviewing or designing an AAC service.

DOI: 10.4324/9781003412311-1

1

WHAT IS AAC AND WHO USES IT?

Helen Robinson

- Words to describe AAC
- Words to describe people
- Using language to empower AAC users and their families
- Who might use AAC?
- Presume competence
- Readiness for AAC
- Common diagnoses where AAC might help
  Intersectionality
- Developmental diagnoses
  Autism
  Cerebral palsy
  Deaf and hard of hearing
  Learning disability
  Rett syndrome
  Situational/selective mutism
  Speech sound disorders and childhood apraxia of speech
- Acquired conditions
  Brain injury
  Guillain-Barré syndrome
  Huntington's disease
  Motor neurone disease
  Multiple sclerosis
  Multiple system atrophy

DOI: 10.4324/9781003412311-2

Primary progressive aphasia

Progressive supranuclear palsy

- Summary
- References

Words to describe AAC

The world of Augmentative and Alternative Communication (AAC) is one filled with jargon. Before we can consider who might benefit from AAC, it's helpful to consider what this term means:

Augmentative is used to describe strategies which support spoken communication. **Alternative** describes strategies which might be used instead of speech.

The International Society for Augmentative and Alternative Communication (ISAAC) offers the following definition:

> AAC is a set of tools and strategies that an individual uses to solve everyday communication challenges. Communication can take many forms such as: speech, a shared glance, text, gestures, facial expressions, touch, sign language, symbols, pictures, **speech generating devices**, etc.
>
> *(ISAAC website, 2023)*

The definition offered by ISAAC could be said to accurately describe the ways in which most of us communicate; nobody relies solely on one single way of communicating; everyone's communication is **multimodal**. However, we are not all **AAC users**.

When we talk about AAC users, we are broadly referring to people who cannot rely on speech to communicate their message some or all of the time and who perhaps use multimodal communication in a unique way (Smith and Jagoe, 2016).

The terms **aided** and **unaided communication** can be used to attempt to describe the different types of AAC (von Tetzchner and Stadskleiv, 2016).

Unaided communication includes speech, vocalisations, gesture, eye-pointing, facial expression.

Aided communication/language includes writing, graphic symbols, voice output **communication aids**/speech generating devices.

Any external tool that a person uses to support their spoken language might be described as a communication aid. Literature referring to those who use aided language will also use the term **aided communicators**, however it's worth noting that these terms are not commonly used by AAC users.

Communication aids have historically been described as "high tech", "mid tech or light tech" and "low tech".

High tech: communication aids which have a touch screen and synthesised voice.

Mid tech or light tech: communication aids which have a recorded voice output and printed overlay.

Low tech: communication aids using printed resources, such as a **graphic symbol** book.

While still in common use, these terms have come under criticism over the years for promoting a linear progression of AAC use, creating expectation that a person will start with low tech and progress through mid to high tech. The terms "high" and "low" could be said to give greater status to one mode of communication over another (Robinson, 2018). The terms **powered AAC** and **paper-based AAC** have become common place and are used throughout this book in place of high tech and low tech, respectively.

Communication aids which have speech output, either via a recorded voice or a synthesised one, are often called "Speech Generating Devices" (SGDs) or "**Voice Output communication Aids" (VOCAs)** in the literature and by practitioners, however AAC users themselves often do not know or like these terms. The term **device** is widely accepted, as is communication device or AAC device. Other terms frequently used are tablet, computer and iPad (even if it isn't an iPad). **Talker** is another term frequently used, however a survey by AssistiveWare (Zisk and Konyn, 2022) highlighted that it is not popular amongst AAC users.

The website of the charity Communication Matters offers an informative booklet explaining what AAC is. The booklet "Other Ways of Speaking" (produced in partnership with Communication Matters, The Communication Trust, 1Voice, ACE Centre, The Makaton

Charity, Scope and Signalong) is available to download for free from www.communicationmatters.org.uk/resources/publications/

Words to describe people

The terms AAC user(s) and **people/person who use AAC** are also used throughout the literature and within the AAC community.

Person first language would support the use of the term *person who uses AAC*. This places emphasis on the person, and not their disability, and has been widely accepted as the preferred choice of language for many years. However, recently there has been a shift towards the use of **identity-first language**, where the disability is identified first, that is, *AAC user*. This term has gained popularity within the AAC community as it destigmatises the use of communication aids, promoting them as a positive aspect of the person's life. There are also people who prefer the term "person who uses AAC". The term **multimodal communicator** is also sometimes used and preferred (Zisk and Konyn, 2022).

People may have a strong opinion about how they would like to be referred to, or they may not have a preference or have given much thought to the terminology. It's always a good idea to ask the person if they have a preference. The term *AAC user* will be used throughout this book.

The terms 'speech' or 'spoken words' are generally accepted as ways to refer to words produced by someone's mouth. The term **mouth words** is gaining popularity. **Non-verbal** has historically been used to describe people who do not use spoken words, but has been criticised for implying that the person doesn't have internal language. The term non-speaking is now frequently used instead (Zisk and Konyn, 2022).

A range of terms might be used to describe the people who work with AAC users. The term professional is frequently used, but some dislike this term as it suggests that the AAC users and their support network are perhaps *un*professional and perpetuates the idea of a hierarchy or **expert model**, where the professional knows best and has power over decisions.

The word clinician might be used, but some feel this is too closely related to the medical model of disability which pathologises people as needing to be "cured" or "fixed".

The term practitioner is perhaps better suited to describing the role of those who support AAC users and it is this term that will be used throughout this book.

Using language to empower AAC users and their families

Much of the terminology used to describe AAC is unfamiliar to the general public, and attempts have been made over the past five decades to suggest alternative vocabulary in an attempt to make AAC more understandable and accessible.

Jo Holmes is a former speech and language therapist (SLT) and parent to Lucy who uses AAC. She writes a wonderful blog about her experiences of AAC called "Mummy Vs. AAC". In a blog post titled "AAC Terminology and Finding a Community of Support" (7 March 2023), Jo agrees that the term AAC can be problematic, however, families of disabled children are well used to acronyms and will likely accept AAC without issue. Additionally, this term is entrenched in the information available online and in the literature, and without an awareness of the term AAC families are unable to search for the help they might need. Jo urges us to use the term AAC "widely, loudly and proudly" (Holmes, 2023).

Who might use AAC?

It is known that 0.5% of the population will benefit from using AAC (Down and Reeves, 2011). AAC can benefit anyone who can't get their message across effectively using speech. The terms non-verbal and non-speaking might often be used to describe AAC users, however, these terms do not reflect the fact that many people who might use AAC will often also use vocalisations or spoken words (Glennen, 1997). People who use communication aids will communicate the majority of their message through other modalities, such as vocalisation and gesture (Clarke, 2016).

People might need to use AAC temporarily, some of the time but not all of the time or lifelong. Those who use AAC some of the time might be referred to as "semi-speaking".

Presume competence

The term presume competence is widely used to describe the belief that any person is capable of learning to use AAC and should have access to it, without the need to prove their abilities first. Presuming competence rejects the idea that there are prerequisite skills for using aided language, instead of testing competence, practitioners are encouraged to seek ways to reveal it (Amanda Hartmann, AssistiveWare blog).

While it seems unimaginable to debate whether someone should or should not be given access to aided language, practitioners working in funded services must also be able to make decisions about what type of support to provide, and when to do this. Funded services must have referral criteria, and once a person has been referred to a service there will be limits as to the amount of support that can be provided. These constraints may therefore not always align with the principle of presuming competence, which can be challenging both to the service users, their families and the practitioners working in these services.

Travers and Ayers (2015) offer a critique of the presume competence movement, which has been rapidly adopted across the wider field of developmental disabilities, especially autism, since the 1990s (Biklen, 1992). Despite early advocates of presuming competence claiming it preserves the dignity of disabled people, no empirical research has been carried out to investigate this.

The presume competence movement is closely linked to the practice of **facilitated communication**, where a person selects letters, words, pictures or objects, often with physical support from another person (the facilitator). Facilitated communication has been researched and shown to be harmful and should not be used (American Speech-Language-Hearing Association (ASHA), 2018). Travers and Ayers suggest that to presume competence is "hazardous" and "minimizes the dignity of the student" (p. 384). They warn against the "false dichotomy" (p. 376) argument which offers only two polar viewpoints; either you believe the person is competent or incompetent. To not presume competence does not mean we assume incompetence. Instead, they encourage us to adopt an agnostic stance and seek evidence of a person's abilities before deciding on how best to support someone.

Comprehensive, personalised assessment along with an understanding of the most current evidence base will support decision making when deciding if and when AAC might be helpful to someone, as described by Alison Felton, SLT, in Box 1.1.

BOX 1.1 A PERSONAL EXPERIENCE OF PRESUMING COMPETENCE

Presume competence' is a term I often use with the adults surrounding a child in order to keep people engaged and active in looking for change and recovery particularly in the acute phase following brain injury. When a child has been in an acute setting for some time with very little change observed it is important to keep everyone looking for that change and presume that the child will be able to access something (and can understand you even when there is little external evidence of response). However, this needs to be managed in terms of expectations. Often hi-tech systems are seen as a sort of 'gold standard' of AAC and a child using eye gaze for play does not mean that it will automatically translate into communication. Focus can be on getting the device to the child through funding etc. but the groundwork by SLTs and others can be extensive prior to this stage and has great value in establishing the building blocks of communication. It can be tremendously disappointing when a child does not really get off the ground with a hi-tech device and it does not develop their communication beyond what they would have established with more basic systems such as choosing from two photographs of objects. So yes, presume competence with caveats.

Alison Felton, SLT

Readiness for AAC

Another term often used is readiness for AAC. This describes whether or not it is the right time to introduce aided language, rather than whether a person meets any prerequisites.

Just as it is important not to delay AAC support, it is also important to recognise the signs that a person, family or setting might not yet be ready to consider AAC; early is not always best, as Jo Holmes describes in Box 1.2.

BOX 1.2 READINESS FOR AAC

A few years ago, I would have maybe said I wished we'd started with symbols sooner BUT with even further hindsight I think that time just spending time connecting was time well spent. If you'd asked me at the time, I would have said we were using Intensive Interaction but really it was more about connection and coping. The early years were overwhelming.

Jo Holmes, parent and former SLT

Practitioners must recognise the power they have over access to AAC assessment services, both in terms of those using the services, and those referring into them. Public awareness of AAC is limited, and this can result in a delay in people accessing support if they don't know what is available, as explained by Jo Holmes in Box 1.3.

BOX 1.3 AAC AWARENESS WITHIN THE GENERAL PUBLIC

I sought out AAC support and had knowledge from my work as an SLT, so I personally found I was able to get and understand the information. I know that I have friends who are also parents of disabled children who have not had this information. I certainly didn't get it from the SLT we saw in the early years who will have seen all of the local children with complex needs.

Jo Holmes, parent and former SLT

It is important to raise awareness of AAC and provide accessible information, to allow potential AAC users and those supporting them to make an informed choice about when to seek an AAC assessment.

The Ace Centre and Talking Mats have produced a resource to help practitioners consider whether a person might be ready to try AAC:

https://acecentre.org.uk/resources/readiness-for-aac

The next part of this chapter describes some groups of people for which AAC might be helpful.

Common diagnoses where AAC might help

AAC can benefit lots of people. There are however a range of diagnoses that are frequently associated with benefitting from AAC. These have been categorised into developmental and acquired diagnoses, rather than child and adult. Developmental diagnoses are those which have been present since birth. Acquired diagnoses are those which have an onset later in life. This might be sudden (i.e., brain injury) or progressive (e.g., motor neurone disease). Much consideration was given to the use of the term "diagnosis" when writing this chapter and the opinion of AAC users and practitioners was sought. For some people, the term diagnosis is problematic as it implies the need for a solution or for the person to be cured. Autistic people and deaf people might prefer the term "identity": 74% of respondents were happy with the term diagnosis or diagnoses being used for the purpose of this chapter.

A description of each diagnosis is given and the common indicators are listed. If a practitioner is already a specialist in this area (e.g., stroke or autism) then it may seem of little benefit to give so much detail here, however, many practitioners working within the world of AAC may not always have such expertise in all of the diagnoses. It is common for speech and language therapists, or occupational therapists, to specialise in AAC and have a hugely varied caseload with many different diagnoses, some which they have little experience in or may only encounter occasionally. For this reason, an overview of the common diagnoses has been provided.

Key points to consider when assessing someone and supporting them to use AAC are given for each diagnosis. Useful websites and resources are listed. It should be notes that the key points listed for consideration are in addition to the broader principles of a comprehensive AAC assessment, which are outlined in Chapter 5.

There are many people who will benefit from AAC but do not have any diagnosis. Also, there are many rare diagnoses that have not been mentioned here that would likely benefit from AAC and their exclusion from this chapter is not to say that AAC should not be considered. What is most important to remember is that every person is an individual and while a diagnosis will give some clues as to their abilities and challenges, everyone will need a comprehensive assessment of their own personal AAC needs. For people without a diagnosis, the earlier description as to who might benefit from AAC will be most helpful.

Terminology is used to describe speech, language and communication disorders. While this will be familiar to speech and language therapists reading this book, definitions have been provided below to help those who may be less familiar with the terms.

Aphasia: a difficulty with understanding and/or using spoken and written language as a result of brain damage.
Apraxia: difficulty carrying out movements on command.
Dysarthria: difficulty with speech caused by muscle weakness.
Dysphagia: difficulty with swallowing.

Intersectionality

People may have multiple categories of social identity which are at greater risk of experiencing inequalities, such as (but not limited to) race, gender, socio-economic status, disability and sexuality. When people experience two or more of these systems of inequality (for example, being a black transgender woman with a disability), the challenges they experience may be increased.

Practitioners supporting people to use AAC should be aware of intersectionality, along with the likelihood of co-occurring communication difficulties and differences. As Beukelman and Mirenda wrote, "There is no typical person who relies on AAC" (2005, p. 4).

Developmental diagnoses

Autism

Autism is a type of neurodivergence (others include Dyslexia, Dysgraphia and Attention Deficit Hyperactivity Disorder (ADHD)) where a person might have differences in:

- How they experience feelings.
- How they communicate.
- How they learn.
- How they think.

Some characteristics of Autism include;

- **Sensory processing/integration difficulties:** the effective interpretation of sensory input.
- **Masking/camouflaging:** hiding certain traits in order to protest as being more neurotypical.
- **Stimming:** self-stimulating behaviour through the repetition of sounds, words or movements.
- **Monotropism:** the tendency to focus on one topic or interest at any given time.
- **Inertia:** a difficulty starting or stopping tasks.
- **Infodumping:** the tendency to share a large amount of information about a topic.

Sometimes, autism occurs alongside a Learning Disability. It's not uncommon for autistic people to have one or more of the other types of neurodivergence (e.g., dyslexia, ADHD). They may also have anxiety and depression.

Information adapted from the website of Emily Lees, Autistic Speech and Language Therapist (2023a) and The National Autistic Society (2023).

Gestalt language processing theory

Gestalt language processing (GLP) was first proposed by Peters (1977) and the theory was later developed by Prizant (1982) and Blanc (2012). Rather than processing language in an analytical way, first using single words, then short phrases and finally full sentences,

Gestalt language processing theory proposes that some people might learn language by first using chunks of language, known as gestalts. They might then apply this gestalt to lots of different contexts, and it might carry linguistic meaning for them. For example, "up, up and away!" might be used to express excitement, because it has been remembered from the child's trip on an aeroplane which was lots of fun for them.

Blanc (2012) built on the earlier work of Prizant (1982), proposing six stages of gestalt language processing, which she described as Natural Language Acquisition (NLA), with **echolalia** being the first stage of language development. Children might then go on to mitigate (break down) this echolalia, where they will add new words to their existing phrases (gestalts). They may then begin to use word combinations, and then progress to applying grammatical rules.

Gestalt language processing theory has recently been criticised for lack of empirical research and for suggesting that autistic people are likely to use GLP (Hutchins, Knox and Fletcher, 2024). There is not currently any research into GLP and AAC use, therefore we are currently unable to confidently say how we might determine if a person uses GLP, or what the best support strategies for AAC users might be. Current clinical experience suggests that the following strategies might be helpful:

- If the person uses spoken **delayed echolalia**, or responds positively to spoken phrases or songs, we should include these on their communication aid.
- Using a voice recording of the phrases, rather than synthesised speech, might be more motivating to the person.
- **Visual scenes** (see Chapter 5) might be beneficial.
- Providing vocabulary that can be used to mitigate the person's gestalts may support their language development. For example, if they say "we gotta go now!" we could provide them with words like "run", "play" or "eat" and encourage phrases like "we gotta go eat!" or "we gotta go play!"

This is a very new field of work and further research is undoubtedly required.

Key points to consider for AAC assessment and support

- Helping an Autistic person to manage their feelings and anxiety, known as sensory regulation, should be a key consideration for any communication support. See The Zones of Regulation Framework (Kuypers, 2011) for further information. AAC might be used to support regulation, either through asking for support ("it's too loud") or stimming (repeating a word over and over to calm themselves).

- The Picture Exchange Communication System (PECS) has widely been used with autistic people for the past three decades. It uses behaviour modification, or operant conditioning, to encourage certain communicative behaviours. A person is encouraged to exchange a picture for a highly motivating item. The autistic community is beginning to reject the use of PECS because it uses physical prompting (see Chapter 6 for more on the prompt hierarchy), can be distressing to the person and communication functions are limited. This is a relatively new shift in thinking, and currently PECS is still widely promoted (Lees, 2023b).
- Consider if the person might be learning language through whole phrases or single words. Provide **core vocabulary, fringe vocabulary** and phrases on their AAC.
- Accessing the internet and photos can support a person's communication and should be available where policy allows.

Useful websites and resources

The Meaningful Speech website has information on Gestalt Language Processing and online courses, including one specific to AAC and GLP:

www.meaningfulspeech.com/AAC-course

Cerebral palsy

Cerebral palsy (CP) affects muscle control and movement and is usually caused by a brain injury before, during or after birth. Children might be delayed in reaching developmental milestones and have a range of motor difficulties. There are three types of CP and people may have a mixture:

Spastic cerebral palsy, characterised by tight muscle tone and stiffness.

Dyskinetic cerebral palsy, characterised by uncontrolled, involuntary muscle spasms (dystonia).

Ataxic cerebral palsy, characterised by coordination difficulties and problems with balance and spatial awareness.

Some conditions associated with cerebral palsy include:

- Visual impairment
- Hearing impairment

- Dysphagia
- Epilepsy
- Periventricular leukomalacia (damage to the brain near the cerebral ventricles)

Key points to consider for AAC assessment and support

- Because CP affects people in a broad range of ways, individual assessment is key.
- People with CP may take a variety of medications to help with their symptoms, and these can impact on their access to AAC both throughout the day and over longer periods. For example;
  - Botox injections might be used to relax the muscles, leading to better control of their arms and hands to access AAC. As the Botox wears off, the person may find their limbs tighten and they need an alternative way of controlling AAC.
  - Certain medications used to treat dystonia can cause the pupils to dilate and impact on the use of eye tracking technology.
  - Medications used to control saliva productions, such as hyoscine patches, can also affect pupil dilation and impact on the use of eye tracking technology.
- When children have severe motor and/or coordination difficulties, eye pointing might often be thought of as a likely means of controlling communication aids. However, it is important to complete a detailed assessment of how the person uses their eye movements prior to considering this as an access method. Some key studies have investigated clinical decision making regarding the use of eye pointing with children with cerebral palsy (Clarke et al., 2022; Griffiths et al., 2023).
- The Eyes on Communication Research Group have carried out several projects. A Delphi study (a process where experts in a given subject are given statements and asked to reach a consensus view) identified issues unique to eye gaze technology and children with Cerebral Palsy (Karlsson et al., 2021). The statements used in the study were then used to develop clinical guidelines, which can be accessed via the website listed.
- Clarke et al. (2020) investigated the use of eye pointing in children with Cerebral Palsy in their "FunVis" project. They have produced a simple, rapid assessment tool to assess the functional vision of children with cerebral palsy. This can be downloaded from the website listed.
- Clarke et al. (2020) have also produced a five-point eye-pointing classification scale (eyepoint scale) which can be used to describe gaze behaviour. This scale can be downloaded from the website listed. It is also available to download as an app for Android and Apple phones.

- Posture, positioning and seating play a big role in how a person might access a communication aid. Involvement of an occupational therapist and/or physiotherapist is important.

Useful websites and resources

Scope:

www.scope.org.uk/
Eye-gaze control technology for people with cerebral palsy – Clinical Guidelines: www.ausacpdm.org.au/resources/eye-gaze-control-technology-for-people-with-cerebral-palsy-2021-clinical-guidelines/
UCL Vision and Communication Research:
www.ucl.ac.uk/gaze/
UCL Rapid Assessment of Functional near Vision:
www.ucl.ac.uk/gaze/funvis
UCL eyepoint classification scale:
www.ucl.ac.uk/gaze/eye-pointing-classification

Deaf and hard of hearing

Deaf and hard of hearing people may use many forms of AAC. In the Deaf community, manual sign languages, such as British Sign Language (BSL), are widely used. These languages have their own word order (syntax) which differs from English. It has been argued that manual sign languages are not a form of unaided AAC, as they are sometimes described, as doing so is ableist and defines them as being less than spoken words (Ofori-Sanzo and Kelly, 2023).

Other sign systems are used, such as Makaton or Sign Supported English (SSE), but it is important to mention that these are not languages, as they are used alongside spoken English, using the same word order. Makaton signs are also represented as graphic symbols. Typically, Makaton is used with children who have a Learning Disability and/or speech sound difficulties, and is not frequently used in the Deaf community.

Children who are deaf or hard of hearing are likely to have a co-occurring diagnosis (approximately 52%), such as a language disorder, learning disability or cerebral palsy (Davies et al., 2009). For these children, manual signing may be delayed or disordered (Morgan, Herman and Woll, 2007, citied in Grove and Launomen, 2019).

Key points to consider for AAC assessment and support

- Co-occurring diagnoses can compound the communication challenges faced by the person and individual assessment is vital (Davies et al., 2009 and von Tetzchner, 2019).
- The default mode of AAC for those with a diagnosis of deafness or hard of hearing is often manual signing. Sensory processing differences or motor sequencing difficulties associated with co-occurring conditions such as dyspraxia or autism can impact a person's success with manual signing. Practitioners must consider the whole person and which mode of AAC might benefit them (von Tetzchner, 2019).
- It has also been observed that sometimes co-occurring conditions, such as a Learning Disability, can be given greater attention than the diagnosis of deafness or hard of hearing and the teaching of manual signing can be overlooked (Gove and Launonen, 2021).
- It is important to consider multimodal communication and explore the preferences of each person, accounting for any linguistic, motor and cognitive difficulties they have. Frequently one mode of aided communication is selected for someone with a diagnosis of deafness or hard of hearing where several different modes might actually be beneficial (Davies et al., 2009; Grove and Launonen, 2019).
- For some people, they may not hear the voice output of a powered communication aid and therefore have greater breakdowns in communication or fail to notice if their communication aid isn't working (Davies et al., 2009).

Useful websites and resources

Royal National Institute for Deaf People (RNID): Information on Technology and assistive devices: https://rnid.org.uk/information-and-support/technology-and-products/

Learning disability

Learning disability is a reduced intellectual ability and difficulty with everyday activities. Learning disability is often described as mild, moderate, severe or profound (referred to as profound and multiple learning disability or PMLD).

Learning disability is different to a learning difficulty, which is a term covering a variety of specific learning needs such as dyslexia, dyscalculia or dysgraphia. A person can have both a learning disability and learning difficulties. A person might have another diagnosis alongside a learning disability, such as Down syndrome or autism (Mencap, 2023).

Key points to consider for AAC assessment and support

- As the term learning disability covers such a broad range of abilities, a comprehensive assessment of the person's speech, language and communication needs is essential.
- As learning disabilities vary in terms of the way they impact a person's communication skills, various forms of AAC might be beneficial to support both receptive and expressive language skills.
- Learning to use AAC can take time and modelling (see Chapter 6) will play a vital role in the success of AAC.

Useful websites and resources

Mencap: www.mencap.org.uk/learning-disability-explained/communicating-people-learning-disability

www.mencap.org.uk/learning-disability-explained/communicating-people-learning-disability/makaton

Rett syndrome

Rett syndrome is a rare neurological disorder caused by a difference on a gene found in the X chromosome and affects more females than males. Children may often follow developmental milestones during the first year and then show a regression of skills between age one and two. Generally, between age two and ten, children's skills will plateau and remain fairly stable for several years. This is then followed by a period of deterioration in movement which might last for many years.

Characteristics include:

- Epilepsy
- Muscle stiffness and/or wastage
- Teeth grinding
- Repetitive hand movements
- Sleep difficulties
- Development of scoliosis (curvature of the spine)
- Apraxia.

(Rett UK, 2023)

Key points to consider for AAC assessment and support

- Some people with Rett syndrome will have an additional learning disability, but not all.
- Apraxia means that access to AAC can be challenging. For most people, eye gaze will be the preferred way to access AAC.
- Rett UK have produced a set of guidelines for supporting communication which can be accessed via the website below.

Useful websites and resources

Rett UK:

www.rettuk.org

Rett UK Communication Professionals Network: www.rettuk.org/resources/resources-for-professionals/rett-uk-speech-language-therapy-network-membership-is-free/

Situational/selective mutism

Situational or selective mutism (SM) is an anxiety-based disorder which impacts a person's ability to speak in certain situations or with certain people. There will be times where they are able to speak without any difficulty. There isn't a strong evidence base for people with SM and the use of AAC (Wilson, 2019).

The consensus is that if a person is anxious to communicate through speaking, they will also be unlikely to communicate through AAC. However, if a person is comfortable using technology, they may find using a powered communication aid easier than speaking in some situations.

Some autistic people might experience periods or situations when they are unable to use speech and will rely on AAC. The term 'semi-speaking' might be preferable for autistic people rather than situational or situational mutism.

Key points to consider for AAC assessment and support

- Be open with those supporting the person, AAC may not be the solution, but it may be worth trying.
- Use Talking Mats (see Chapter 4) to gain the person's opinion about if and when they might want to explore using AAC.

Useful websites and resources

SMiRA (Selective Mutism Information & Research Association): www.selectivemutism.org.uk/

CALL Scotland have a blog post which offers some anecdotal advice about SM and links to research:

www.callscotland.org.uk/blog/selective-mutism-and-technology/

Speech sound disorders and childhood apraxia of speech

Speech sound disorders is a term used to describe a developmental difficulty with articulation (forming clear speech sounds), phonology (sequences or patterns of sound) and prosody (stress, intonation and volume). Other terms may also be used, such as dyspraxia, childhood apraxia of speech (CAS) and developmental verbal dyspraxia (DVD). There has been a gradual shift towards using the term Childhood Apraxia of Speech (Broomfield, Cleland and Williams, 2023).

Speech and Language Therapy can help and most children go on to develop intelligible speech, however there is a small population who will experience ongoing difficulties producing clear speech.

Speech sound disorders may occur in isolation, or alongside some other characteristics including:

- Receptive and expressive language difficulties
- Autism
- Difficulty with language organisation, particularly sequencing
- Generalised Developmental Coordination Disorder (CDC/Dyspraxia)

(Dyspraxia Foundation, 2023)

Key points to consider for AAC assessment and support

- People will generally show a preference for using speech, even if it is highly unintelligible. Even if those supporting them can see the benefit of AAC, it's very common for people with speech sound disorders to persist with their speech.
- Some people may not be aware of their level of unintelligibility and not see the value of AAC.

- Younger children will often cope very well without AAC, especially when in a supporting environment with adults who are in-tune with their communication skills. This can make introducing communication aids very challenging as it may be seen as a "task" which is required of them. Modelling the use of AAC can help (see Chapter 6).
- People may use AAC occasionally to support their speech. They might not benefit from AAC based around core words, but instead do well with something based around topic vocabulary or key phrases.
- It can be challenging to predict the words the person might need in their aided language system and therefore providing them with descriptive words can be beneficial. They can use these words to describe the attributes of the word they are trying to communicate, rather than searching for a specific word which might not be available on their communication aid.
- Training the communication partner to ask appropriate questions to support communication breakdowns can be very beneficial.

Useful websites and resources

The Dyspraxia Foundation:

https://dyspraxiafoundation.org.uk/professionals_pages/speech-and-language/

Afasic:

www.afasic.org.uk/slcn/

Acquired conditions

Brain injury

There are different types of brain injury and many causes. The main causes are listed below:

- Traumatic brain injury (head injury)
- Brain tumours
- Stroke
- Brain haemorrhage
- Encephalitis
- Brain aneurysm

- Carbon monoxide poisoning
- Hydrocephalus
- Hypoxic and anoxic brain injury
- Meningitis.

(Headway, 2023)

Because brain injuries are so varied, the effects are wide ranging. The symptoms which are likely to impact AAC use are listed below, but there are many more possible effects of brain injury:

- Behavioural and emotional changes
- Cognitive changes and memory problems
- Executive dysfunction
- Fatigue
- Physical difficulties
- Aphasia
- Dysarthria
- Dyspraxia
- Attention and concentration difficulties
- Reduced reasoning and problem-solving skills
- Slower processing skills
- Reduced insight

When the brain injury occurs in the brain stem, this can cause total paralysis of all muscles except for vertical eye movement, known a "Locked-in syndrome".

Key points to consider for AAC assessment and support

- The cognitive changes associated with brain injury can mean learning to use AAC can be challenging.
- In cases of locked-in syndrome, cognitive function is not usually affected. AAC will need to utilise an "up-down" eye movement as an access method.
- Assessment of a person's vision can be a key aspect of assessment.
- Colour coding can help people understand the organisation of AAC vocabularies, e.g., question words, people words. See Chapter 5 for further details.
- It is important to assess literacy skills to build a detailed picture of the person's abilities.
- Word finding problems present in spoken language will also likely be present in AAC use. It's vital to investigate the person's semantic skills before thinking about AAC.

- Organisation of the vocabulary can impact on how well AAC is used. People with impaired semantic skills may struggle with vocabulary being organised **taxonomically** and benefit from **schematic organisation** and/or visual scenes. The context of the visual scenes can matter greatly and thorough assessment is required. See chapter five for further information.

Useful websites and resources

The charity Headway has a website with an extensive amount of information and resources: https://www.headway.org.uk/

Guillain-Barré syndrome

Guillain-Barré syndrome (GBS) is a rare auto-immune disease which causes damage to the peripheral nervous system, usually (but not always) caused by the immune system over-reacting to an infection. It affects around one to two people per 100,000 each year and adult males are more likely to be diagnosed, although it can also occur in females and children.

GBS causes inflammation of the myelin of the neurones, preventing brain signals from being sent effectively and resulting in pain, numbness and weakness in the limbs. Onset is often sudden and symptoms progress rapidly over the course of a few weeks, reaching the severest within two to four weeks. Early symptoms include pins and needles, muscle weakness, coordination difficulties and numbness. Later symptoms of GBS include:

- Difficulty walking
- Paralysis
- Difficulty breathing
- Speech loss
- Dysphagia
- Bowel problems
- Severe pain
- Facial weakness

Most people with GBS will make a good recovery, although this can take many months and some people will be left with longer-term symptoms. GBS can result in death for around 2–5% of people. There are several variations of GBS, which may cause the person to present with differing combinations of motor and sensory symptoms and/or decreased consciousness (GAIN Charity, 2023).

Key points to consider for AAC assessment and support

- Loss of speech is likely to be sudden. People with GBS are likely to present in acute medical settings. GBS may not be diagnosed immediately and the lack of information can be distressing to the person and those close to them.
- Receptive language is not impacted, although people may be sedated which may impact how responsive they are.
- Some people may experience visual disturbances which might impact on their use of AAC. It might be difficult to know that they are experiencing this.
- Speech may continue to worsen over time.
- The way in which a person accesses AAC may need to change as the disease progresses and then later improves.
- The person's family may need to be consulted to help gather a history of their previous communication skills to help inform AAC choices, for example, whether the person can use the alphabet to communicate. It's important not to assume prior literacy skills.

Useful websites and resources

GAIN (Guillain-Barré and Associated Inflammatory Neuropathies)

www.gaincharity.org.uk

Huntington's disease

Huntington's disease is a genetic condition inherited from one or both parents. It is a progressive neurological disorder. Symptoms usually appear between ages 30 and 50, but can occur in childhood. If onset is before 20 years old it is called Juvenile Huntington's disease. The symptoms of Huntington's disease are:

- Motor difficulties, including jerky, involuntary movements
- Cognitive difficulties including memory loss, concentration problems and mood changes
- Depression and personality changes
- Difficulty with swallowing and breathing
- Dysarthria impacting clarity of speech
- Word finding difficulties
- Receptive language difficulties

Symptoms worsen over a period of 20 years, eventually resulting in death (Huntington's Disease Association, 2023; Bachoud-Lévi et al., 2019).

Key points to consider for AAC assessment and support

- Symptoms and rate of progression will vary within individuals and communication assessment and review will be ongoing. Support will also need to vary and respond to the needs of the individual.
- Cognitive difficulties frequently impact a person's ability to learn and remember how to use AAC, therefore early support is important.
- The cognitive changes are likely to have a significant impact on the person's communication skills. People often become apathetic and not interested in learning to use AAC.
- Depression, mood and personality changes can affect a person's social interaction and motivation to communicate. People often become withdrawn.
- Motor difficulties will likely impact how a person can access AAC and this will change as the disease progresses. Learning new ways to access AAC can be challenging for the person.
- If the person was literate before the onset of their symptoms, it is likely they will lose these skills over time and will need to use graphic symbols for communication.
- It is important to train the person's communication partners to be able to support their changing communication needs (Bachoud-Lévi et al., 2019; Hamilton et al., 2012).

Useful websites and resources

The Huntington's Disease Association:

www.hda.org.uk/

Huntington's disease: Behaviour and communication guide:

www.hda.org.uk/media/2517/behaviour-and-communication-guide.pdf

Motor neurone disease

Motor neurone disease (MND) is perhaps the most well-known of the neurodegenerative conditions but is still considered to be rare. Like others, it attacks the neurones and affects the brain's ability to control the body. MND is progressive and life limiting. It generally affects people over the age of 50 but can affect younger adults too. There are four types:

Amyotrophic lateral sclerosis (ALS): This is the most common type of MND. Life expectancy is two to five years from onset of symptoms.

Bulbar onset MND or Progressive bulbar palsy (PBP): This mostly affects the muscles of the face, throat and tongue, so speech difficulties are often the first symptom. Life expectancy is between six months and three years from onset of symptoms.

Progressive muscular atrophy (PMA): This is a rarely seen type of MND, characterised by weakness in the hands initially. Life expectancy is usually beyond five years.

Primary Lateral sclerosis (PLS): This is a rare form of MND, where a person's lower limbs are affected first. PLS is usually not life shortening as it progresses very slowly.

Symptoms include:

- Muscle weakness, cramps and spasms
- Dysarthria
- Dysphagia
- Breathing problems and difficulty coughing
- Emotional lability
- Mild cognitive changes (about half of people)
- A small number of people may develop frontotemporal dementia.

(MNDA, 2023)

Key points to consider for AAC assessment and support

- People with MND may wish to explore voice and message banking, but not everyone wants to do this. It's important to have this conversation as early as possible.
- The progressive nature of the disease means that the type of AAC will change, sometimes rapidly. A person may begin by using their hands to access AAC and later require alternative **access methods** such as switch scanning or eye tracking technology.
- Cognitive changes may impact a person's ability to learn how to use AAC.
- Breathing difficulties may mean a person has to wear a full or partial face mask if they are ventilated. This can mean eye pointing or eye gaze technology is challenging.

Useful websites and resources

The motor neurone disease association has a fabulous range of resources for practitioners: www.mndassociation.org/professionals/

The MNDA can support people in the UK to access communication aids by providing financial support or equipment loans. They will also support with **voice banking**, by providing equipment for this and advice:

www.mndassociation.org/support-and-information/our-services/communication-aids-service/

Multiple sclerosis

Multiple sclerosis (MS) is a neurological condition affecting the central nervous system. It occurs more frequently in women than men and onset of symptoms usually occurs between age 20 and 40. MS is an autoimmune and neurodegenerative condition, where the immune system attacks the myelin of the nerve cells causing difficulties with the brain sending signals to parts of the body. It is not fatal. Symptoms vary greatly between individuals and there are three types:

Relapsing remitting: This accounts for 85% of MS diagnoses. People will have periods when symptoms suddenly worsen (a relapse), followed by a period of recovery (remission).

Secondary progressive: People may initially be diagnosed with relapsing remitting MS then find that over time, they stop having the periods of remission and their symptoms continue to progress.

Primary progressive: People experience a constant progression in their symptoms from the onset, without any periods of remission.

Symptoms include:

- Fatigue
- Pins and needles, numbness or burning sensation of the skin
- Problems with eye sight, including blurred vision
- Cognitive changes
- Movement difficulties
- Muscle stiffness and spasms
- Problems with balance and coordination

Key points to consider for AAC assessment and support

- Symptoms and rate of progression will vary within individuals and communication assessment and review will be ongoing. Support will also need to vary and respond to the needs of the individual.

- Motor difficulties will likely impact how a person can access AAC and this will change as the disease progresses. Learning new ways to access AAC can be challenging for the person.
- Cognitive changes can make learning new skills challenging. A person might have difficulty processing information about AAC and find it hard to generalise and maintain new skills.
- Fatigue can impact a person's participation in therapy sessions.
- Vision difficulties can mean using eye tracking technology isn't possible for some people. It's worth considering a **head mouse** if they have good control of their head movements.

Useful websites and resources

The Multiple Sclerosis Trust (UK) has an excellent range of resources for Speech and Language Therapists:

https://mstrust.org.uk/a-z/speech-and-language-therapy

Multiple system atrophy

Multiple system atrophy (MSA) is a rare neurodegenerative disorder, previously known as Shy-Drager syndrome, with no known genetic or environmental cause. Presentation is similar to Parkinson's, with both conditions primarily affecting motor skills, however there are a few key differences. Onset of symptoms is usually earlier than with Parkinson's, occurring at around age 50. Multiple areas of the brain will be affected, including the cerebellum (balance and coordination) and the autonomic nervous system (blood pressure, body temperature, urination, sexual function).

There are two types of MSA and individuals can vary in terms of presentation, often with mixed symptoms that change over time. Progression ranges between five and 20 years, but most people will die within six to ten years of the onset of symptoms (The MSA Coalition, 2023).

MSA-predominant Parkinsonism (MSA-P). This is the most common type of MSA

- Movement difficulties, often with muscle rigidity
- Resting tremor
- Dysarthria

- Voice changes
- Dysphagia
- Dysautonomia (dysfunction of the automatic nervous system) affecting blood pressure, breathing and digestion
- Cognitive impairment is present in some cases of MSA; however, the literature reports wide ranging incidence and is inconclusive

MSA-predominant cerebellar ataxia (MSA-C)

- Coordination difficulties affecting walking, hand movements, eye movements.
- Dysarthria.

Key points to consider for AAC assessment and support

- Symptoms and rate of progression will vary within individuals and communication assessment and review will be ongoing. Support will also need to vary and respond to the needs of the individual.
- Motor difficulties will likely impact how a person can access AAC and this will change as the disease progresses. Learning new ways to access AAC can be challenging for the person.
- Cognitive impairment may occur, and impact communication skills including previous literacy skills. AAC may progress from keyboard spelling, to whole word phrases and sometimes graphic symbols.

Useful websites and resources

The MSA Coalition

www.multiplesystematrophy.org/

Parkinson's UK

www.parkinsons.org.uk/

Primary progressive aphasia

Primary progressive aphasia (PPA) is a neurodegenerative condition caused by other conditions such as Alzheimer's disease or frontotemporal lobar degeneration. A person's language skills become progressively impaired over time, often resulting in the person being unable to understand and use spoken or written language. Other symptoms associated with the underlying condition may also be present, such as memory loss. Because PPA is associated with other conditions and neurological degeneration, the symptoms and progression will vary from person to person.

PPA can be classified as three distinct types:

- **Semantic dementia:** Characterised by difficulties with words finding or remembering the use of everyday household items. Receptive language skills will decline, along with literacy. The person my talk at length about the same thing. Behaviour and personality changes are common.
- **Progressive non-fluent aphasia:** Characterised by mistakes with spoken words, stammering, slower or quieter speech. Word order and grammar is likely to be affected, along with receptive language. Literacy skills will be impaired. Other symptoms include hearing loss, dysphagia, behaviour and mood changes. People may experience motor difficulties, such as shaking and balance problems.
- **Logopenic aphasia:** Characterised by word finding difficulties and dysfluent speech. Receptive language and memory are also impaired.

(Alzheimer's Research UK, 2023)

Key points to consider for AAC assessment and support

- AAC can benefit people with PPA, however as speech, language and communication skills continue to deteriorate the type of AAC the person uses will need to change and may eventually not be useful for them at all.
- Because a person's receptive language and word finding skills are affected, their ability to search for words in an **AAC system** will also be impaired.
- A person may start off with text based AAC and then change to graphic symbol communication.

Useful websites and resources

Alzheimer's Research UK:

www.alzheimersresearchuk.org/dementia-information/types-of-dementia/primary-progressive-aphasia/

National Aphasia Association:

www.aphasia.org/aphasia-resources/primary-progressive-aphasia/

Progressive supranuclear palsy

Progressive supranuclear palsy (PSP) is a rare neurodegenerative disorder, affecting coordination, eye movements, speech and cognition. It may also be known as Steele-Richardson-Olszewski syndrome. Average age of onset is age 60 but can occur from 40 onwards.

Symptoms include:

- Difficulty with balance and motor coordination
- Dysarthria
- Dysphagia
- Aphasia
- Ataxia
- Paralinguistic changes (speech volume and rate)
- Cognitive changes, especially in mood and personality
- Changes in eye movements, especially looking up and down due to paralysis of the muscles that move the eyeballs.

(Cure PSP, February 2023; PSPA, February 2023)

Corticobasal degeneration (CBD) is similar to PSP and the symptoms often overlap. Cognitive changes, such as impulsive behaviour, lack of empathy are often the first symptoms to occur in CBD. People with CBD also often experience numbness on one side of the body (PSPA, February 2023).

Key points to consider for AAC assessment and support

- Symptoms and rate of progression will vary within individuals and communication assessment and review will be ongoing. Support will also need to vary and respond to the needs of the individual.
- Motor difficulties will likely impact how a person can access AAC and this will change as the disease progresses. Learning new ways to access AAC can be challenging for the person.
- Cognitive impairment may occur, and impact communication skills including previous literacy skills. AAC may progress from keyboard spelling, to whole word phrases and sometimes graphic symbols.
- Difficulties with eye movements can impact how a person access AAC. Partner assisted Auditory scanning books can often be very helpful.

Useful websites and resources

PSP Association:

www.psp.org/

Funding for voice banking in the UK:

www.pspassociation.org. https://www.pspassociation.org.uk/information-and-support/for-professionals/resources-for-professionals/uk/information-and-support/pspa-voice-banking/

Information for practitioners supporting people with PSP:

www.pspassociation.org.uk/information-and-support/for-professionals/resources-for-professionals/

Cure PSP

www.psp.org/

Parkinson's UK

www.parkinsons.org.uk/

Summary

AAC might be useful for anyone who can't always get their message across using speech. The terminology used to define and describe AAC can be unfamiliar to the general public and practitioners need to be mindful of this when discussing AAC with people and those who support them. Awareness raising and accessible information is the key to helping people to make informed decisions about accessing AAC services.

There are some diagnoses which are typically associated with AAC use, although not everyone with these diagnoses will benefit from AAC. It's helpful to consider the common symptoms, or characteristics of these diagnoses and reflect on how that might impact our assessment and the support we give people. However, overall, we must remember that people are individuals, and a comprehensive assessment of their abilities, needs and preferences for communication is key.

References

Alzheimer's Research UK (2023, 26 February). Primary progressive aphasia. www.alzheimersresearchuk.org/dementia-information/types-of-dementia/primary-progressive-aphasia/.

American Speech-Language-Hearing Association (ASHA) (2018). Position statement: Facilitated communication. www.asha.org/policy/ps201800352/#:~:text=References,Position%20Statement%3A%20Facilitated%20Communication,that%20should%20not%20be%20used.

Bachoud-Lévi, A. C., Ferreira, J., Massart, R., Youssov, K., Rosser, A., Busse, M., Craufurd, D., Reilmann, R., De Michele, G., Rae, D., Squitieri, F., Seppi, K., Perrine, C., Scherer-Gagou, C., Audrey, O., Verny, C. and Burgunder, J. M. (2019). International guidelines for the treatment of Huntington's disease. *Frontiers in Neurology*, 10(3), 1–18. doi: 10.3389/fneur.2019.00710.

Beukelman, D. R. and Mirenda, P. (2005). *Augmentative & Alternative Communication: Supporting Children & Adults with Complex Communication Needs* (3rd ed.). Taylor & Francis.

Biklen, D. (1992). Communication unbound: Autism and praxis. *Hospital Practice*, 27(4), 209-250. https://doi.org/10.1080/21548331.1992.11705407.

Blanc, M. (with Lyon, J. G.) (2012). *Natural Language Acquisition on the Autism Spectrum: The Journey from Echolalia to Self-generated Language*. Communication Development Center.

Broomfield, J., Cleland, J. and Williams, P. (2023, Winter). What's in a name? *RCSLT Bulletin*, (833), 22-23.

Clarke, M., (2016). Co-construction, asymmetry and multimodality in children's conversations. In M. Smith and J. Murray (eds), *The Silent Partner? Language, Interaction and Aided Communication* (pp. 179–197). J & R Press Ltd.

Clarke, M. T., Sargent, J., Cooper, R., Aberbach, G., McLaughlin, L., Panesar, G., Griffiths, T., Price, K., Rose, C. and Swettenham, J. (2020). Development and testing of the eye-pointing classification scale for children with cerebral palsy. *Disability and Rehabilitation*, 44(8), 1451–1456. https://doi.org/10.1080/09638288.2020.1800834.

Cure PSP (2023, 22 February). What is PSP? www.psp.org/iwanttolearn/progressive-supranuclear-palsy/#page-section-what-is-psp?.

Davies, T. N., Barnard-Brak, L., Dacus, D. and Pond, A. (2009). Aided AAC systems among individuals with hearing loss and disabilities. *Journal or Developmental ad Physical Disabilities*, 22, 241–256, https://doi.org/10.1007/s10882-009-9180-6.

Down, K. and Reeves, A. (2011) Specialised AAC provision - Commissioning national services. Office of the Communication Champion and Council. Communication Matters website (2023, 15 February). www.communicationmatters.org.uk/resources/publications/.

Dyspraxia Foundation (2023, 26 February). What is dyspraxia? https://dyspraxiafoundation.org.uk/what_is_dyspraxia/developmental-verbal-dyspraxia/.

GAIN Charity (2023, 18 February). What is GBS? https://gaincharity.org.uk/faq/gbs-and-acute-associated-inflammatory-neuropathies/.

Glennen, S. L. (1997). Introduction to augmentative and alternative communication. In S. L. Glennen and D. C. DeCoste (eds) *Handbook of Augmentative and Alternative Communication* (pp. 3–20). Tomson Learning.

Griffiths, T., Clarke, M. T., & Swettenham, J. (2023). The ability of typically developing 2-3 year olds to infer the control mechanism for eye-gaze technology and the impact of causal language instruction. *Disability and Rehabilitation: Assistive Technology*, 1–8. https://doi.org/10.1080/17483107.2023.2293874.

Grove, N. and Launonen, K. (2019). Signing in the margins: An introduction. In N. Grove and K. Launonen (eds) *Manual Sign Acquisition in Children with Developmental Disabilities* (pp. 1–19). Nova Science publishers, Inc.

Hartmann, A. (nd). Presuming competence. *AssistiveWare*. www.assistiveware.com/learn-aac/presume-competence.

Hamilton, A., Ferm, U., Heemskerk, A-W., Twiston-Daview, R., Metheson, K. Y., Simpson, S. A. and Rae, D. (2012). Management of speech, language and communication difficulties in Huntington's disease. *Neurodegenerative Disease Management*, 2(1), 67–77. doi: 10.3389/fneur.2019.00710.

Headway (2023, 24 February). About brain injury. www.headway.org.uk/about-brain-injury/.
Holmes, J. (2023, 8 March). *AAC Terminology and finding a community of support*. Mummy vs AAC blog. www.mummyvsaac.blog/aac-terminology-and-finding-a-community-of-support/.
Huntington's Disease Association (2023, 18 February). *Managing communication difficulties*. www.hda.org.uk/getting-help/if-youre-a-carer/managing-communication-difficulties.
Hutchins, T. L., Knox, S. E. and Fletcher, E. C. (2024). Natural language acquisition and gestalt language processing: A critical analysis of their application to autism and speech language therapy. *Autism & Developmental Language Impairments*, *9*. https://doi.org/10.1177/23969415241249944.
ISAAC (2023, 15 February). What is AAC? https://isaac-online.org/english/what-is-aac/.
Karlsson, P., Griffiths, T., Clarke, M. T., Monbaliu, E., Himmelmann., Bekeshi, S., Allsop, A., Pereksles, R., Galea, C. and Wallen, M. (2021). Stakeholder consensus for decision making in eye-gaze control technology for children, adolescents and adults with cerebral palsy provision: Findings from a Delphi study. *BMC Neurology*, 21, 21–63. https://doi.org/10.1186/s12883-021-02077-z.
Kuypers, L. M. (2011). *The Zones of Regulation*. Think Social Publishing.
Lees, E. (2023a, 7 March). What is autism? www.autisticslt.com/whatisautism.
Lees, E. (2023a, 8 March). So what's wrong with PECS? www.autisticslt.com/pecs-aba.
Mencap (2023, 26 February). What is a learning disability? www.mencap.org.uk/learning-disability-explained/what-learning-disability.
Morgan, G., Herman, R. & Woll, B. (2007). Language impairments in sign language: breakthroughs and puzzles. *International Journal of Language & Communication Disorders*, 42(1), pp. 97–105. doi: 10.1080/13682820600783178.
Motor Neurone Disease Association (2023, 24 February). *About MND*. www.mndassociation.org/about-mnd/.
Multiple Sclerosis Trust (2023, 24 February). What is MS? https://mstrust.org.uk/information-support/about-ms/what-is-ms.
National Aphasia Association (2023, 16 February). Primary progressive aphasia. www.aphasia.org/aphasia-resources/primary-progressive-aphasia/.
National Autistic Society (2023, 7 March). What is autism? www.autism.org.uk/advice-and-guidance/what-is-autism.
Ofori-Sanzo, K. and Kelly, Q. [@thesigningslp]. (2023, March 10). Currently, ASHA lists ASL as a form of unaided AAC. Instagram. www.instagram.com/p/CpVbEmoOiDx/?igshid=MDJmNzVkMjY=.
Peters, A. M. (1977). Language learning strategies: Does the whole equal the sum of the parts? *Language*, 560–573.
Prizant, B. M. (1982). Gestalt language and gestalt processing in autism. *Topics in Language Disorders*, 3(1), 16–23.
PSP Association (2023, 22 February). A brief guide to CBD. www.pspassociation.org.uk/information-and-support/what-is-cbd/a-brief-guide-to-cbd/.
PSP Association (2023, 22 February). A brief guide to PSP. www.pspassociation.org.uk/information-and-support/what-is-psp/brief-guide-to-psp/.
Rett UK (2023, 28 February). What is Rett Syndrome? www.rettuk.org/what-is-rett-syndrome/.
RNID (2023, 1 March). Types and causes of hearing loss and deafness. https://rnid.org.uk/information-and-support/hearing-loss/types-of-hearing-loss-and-deafness/noise-induced-hearing-loss/.
Robinson, H. (2018, March). AAC technology: What's in a name? *RCSLT Bulletin*, 11, 791.
Selective Mutism Information & Research Association (SMIRA) (2023, 26 February). About selective mutism. www.selectivemutism.org.uk/.
Scope (2023, 26 February). Cerebral palsy (CP). www.scope.org.uk/advice-and-support/cerebral-palsy-introduction/.
Smith, M. and Jagoe, C. (2016). Relevance in the context of multimodality and aided communication. In M. M. Smith and J. Murray (eds) *The Silent Partner? Language, Interaction and Aided Communication* (pp. 229–246). J & R Press Ltd.

Smith, M. and J. Murray (2016). *The Silent Partner? Language, Interaction and Aided Communication*. J & R Press Ltd.

The MSA Coalition (2023, 22 February). What is multiple system atrophy? www.multiplesystematrophy.org/about-msa/.

Travers, J., Ayres, K. M. (2015). A critique of presuming competence of learners with autism or other developmental disabilities. *Education and Training in Autism and Developmental Disabilities*, 50(4), 371–387.

von Tetzchner, S. (2019). Manual signs and graphic symbols as complementary forms of augmentative and alternative communication. In N. Grove and K. Launonen (eds) *Manual Sign Acquisition in Children with Developmental Disabilities* pp. 195–212. Nova Science publishers, Inc.

Von Tetzchner, S., & Stadskleiv, K. (2016). Constructing a language in alternative forms. In J. Murray & M. M. Smith (Eds.), *The Silent Partner? Language, Interaction and Aided Communication* pp. 17–34. J & R Press Ltd.

Wilson, A. (2019, May 24th)). Selective Mutism and Technology, CALL Scotland blog. https://www.callscotland.org.uk/blog/selective-mutism-and-technology/

Zisk, A. H., & Konyn, Lily. (2022, November). How to talk about AAC and aAAC users (according to them). *AssistiveWare Blog*. https://www.assistiveware.com/blog/how-to-talk-about-aac

2

HOW DO WE CHOOSE WHICH TYPE OF AAC TO USE?

Helen Robinson

- Why decisions matter
- Decision-making models

    The five principles for AAC

    Human Activity Assistive Technology Model

    Matching Person to Technology Model
- I-ASC Explanatory Model of AAC decision making
- What are the decisions that need to be made?
- Who is making the decisions?

    The person

    The family of the person

    Speech and language therapist (SLT)

    Occupational therapist (OT)

    Educational practitioners

    Other practitioners
- Open AAC
- Ways of gathering information

    Asking people

    Observing

    Activities

    The Frenchay screening tool for AAC

    Test of aided communication (TASP)
- AAC assessment observation checklist

DOI: 10.4324/9781003412311-3

- How do we know when we've found the right AAC?
- AAC trial goals
- What to do when there is difference in opinion
- Summary
- AAC trial record form
- References

Why decisions matter

Providing someone with AAC which meets their needs can mean better access to education and employment as well as overall quality of life. Despite these benefits, the rate of abandonment of AAC is high, although we do not clearly understand the reasons why people give up (Webb et al., 2019).

The pressure to make the right decision can be great. Providing someone with AAC which isn't suitable has consequences for both the individual, those supporting them and those that have funded the communication aid. For the individual, being given something which is too difficult to use, doesn't have the right words or isn't reliable might result in them rejecting future trials of communication aids. For those supporting them, being asked to use something which isn't intuitive or which they perceive to be too difficult to learn might negatively impact their attitude towards AAC overall, affecting the support they give to both this individual and others in future. The abandonment of communication aids is costly to those who fund them; therefore, it is important that we understand how and why decisions are made so that we might give each individual the best possible chance of success.

Decision-making models

The five principles for AAC

When choosing AAC, practitioners may wish to consider the five principles for AAC proposed by Williams, Krezman and McNaughton (2008). These principles are based on the published writings of AAC users and their families:

The time for AAC is now

Communication is a basic human right. People who would likely benefit from AAC are still frequently overlooked by practitioners, or may not even have an awareness that AAC is available. Individuals shouldn't have to prove that they are "ready" for AAC before it is offered to them. This idea is often referred to as "presume competence".

One is never enough

Multimodal communication is important, as is having multiple communication partners that understand the strategies the person uses is vital. Having a range of AAC strategies and communication partners that are confident in supporting these will enable the person to communicate across a range of environments.

My AAC must fit my life

The person's AAC will need to be highly individualised in order to make them easy to use and easy to learn. Communication aids should have tools and supports to make them easier to adopt. Communication aids must be appealing to those that use them.

AAC must support full participation in all aspects of 21st-century life

Communication aids must provide people with all the vocabulary they might require to participate fully in their lives as they grow. This includes words for employment, medical appointments, financial decisions and relationships. Without this language the individual loses out on opportunities in life, and society loses out on their valuable contributions. Ongoing support must be available and practitioners must not underestimate the potential of AAC users.

Nothing about me without me

Often, AAC users are not included in the decision-making process. We must both seek and listen to the opinions of AAC users when researching, developing and supporting AAC use. Their lived experiences will provide a valuable insight into the products they are provided with.

Human Activity Assistive Technology Model

Practitioners may understandably look towards models which help them make decisions regarding which AAC to choose.

Bailey (1996) proposed the Human Performance Model (HPM), in which somebody (a person), is doing something (an activity), at some place (within a context). The Human Activity Assistive Technology Model (HAAT) builds on the HPM to include the use of assistive technology, such as powered communication aids. The HAAT model has four factors:

Human factors include:

- Motivation, values and attitude towards AAC
- Confidence
- Involvement in decision making and ownership

Activity factors include:

- The need to communicate across a range of environments
- The opportunities the person has
- Whether or not AAC is seen as part of their routines

Assistive technology factors include:

- Reliability
- How easy it is to generate a message

All of the human, activity and assistive technology factors exist within the context. This includes the support available to the person, the time available and the attitudes of those supporting them.

Matching Person to Technology Model

Marcia Scherer's Matching Person to Technology (MPT) Model (Scherer, 2005) highlights three areas that are likely to impact successful technology use; the person, the environment and the functions and features of the technology (Scherer and Federici, 2015). Factors in the environment might include the support provided, whether the people supporting the person encourage the use of the technology and if the decision was made by someone else. Person characteristics might include the expectations of how much the technology will benefit them, or if they feel self-conscious about using the technology. Technology features might be how comfortable it is to use, if it is too complicated or if the customer support is unreliable (Scherer and Federici, 2015).

The following website offers an assessment tool to support the decision-making process when selecting appropriate technology for a person. This is not AAC specific, but the principles can be applied to powered communication aids: https://sites.google.com/view/matchingpersontechnology/home

I-ASC Explanatory Model of AAC decision making

Webb et al. (2019) describe how despite a lack of rigorous evidence being available to practitioners who are involved in the decision-making process, overall, they are often basing their assessment on the five principles outlined by Williams, Krezman and McNaughton (2008), however, they also highlight the need for better tools to support practitioners to make decisions around AAC.

A three-and-a-half-year research project in the United Kingdom titled "Identifying appropriate symbol communication aids for children who are non-speaking: enhancing clinical decision making" was carried out between 2016–2019. This is also known as "I-ASC – Identifying Appropriate Symbol Communication" or simply "I-ASC study" (pronounced "I ask"). (Lynch et al., 2019; Murray et al., 2019).

The I-ASC study aimed to improve the outcomes for children with little or no intelligible speech who need symbol communication aids to communicate, through the development of resources to the help people make decisions when choosing communication aids, such as health and education practitioners, alongside the AAC user and their family and other key partners.

The research team first used systematic reviews to explore the current evidence, then held focus groups with practitioners who regularly carried out AAC assessments. Next, the opinions of young AAC users were gained via interviews, alongside the opinions of their families and practitioners involved in their assessment. Practitioners were then asked to complete surveys to investigate the factors they considered important when choosing which AAC to provide. The results of this process were used to develop a decision-making resource (also referred to as a heuristic) which would help practitioners, AAC users and their families to consider the different parts of the AAC assessment process. The I-ASC Explanatory Model of AAC decision making is shown in Figure 2.1.

This I-ASC Explanatory Model of AAC decision making (Figure 2.1) shows the three competing considerations in the top three cogs, offering a visual representation of how the child's characteristics, the access features and the communication aid attributes will interlink and how one decision might influence another, causing the cogs to shift and decisions to narrow, as described earlier in this chapter. The descriptors from within each cog can be found at https://iasc.mmu.ac.uk/wp-content/uploads/2019/05/I-ASC-Competing-considerations-descriptors.pdf.

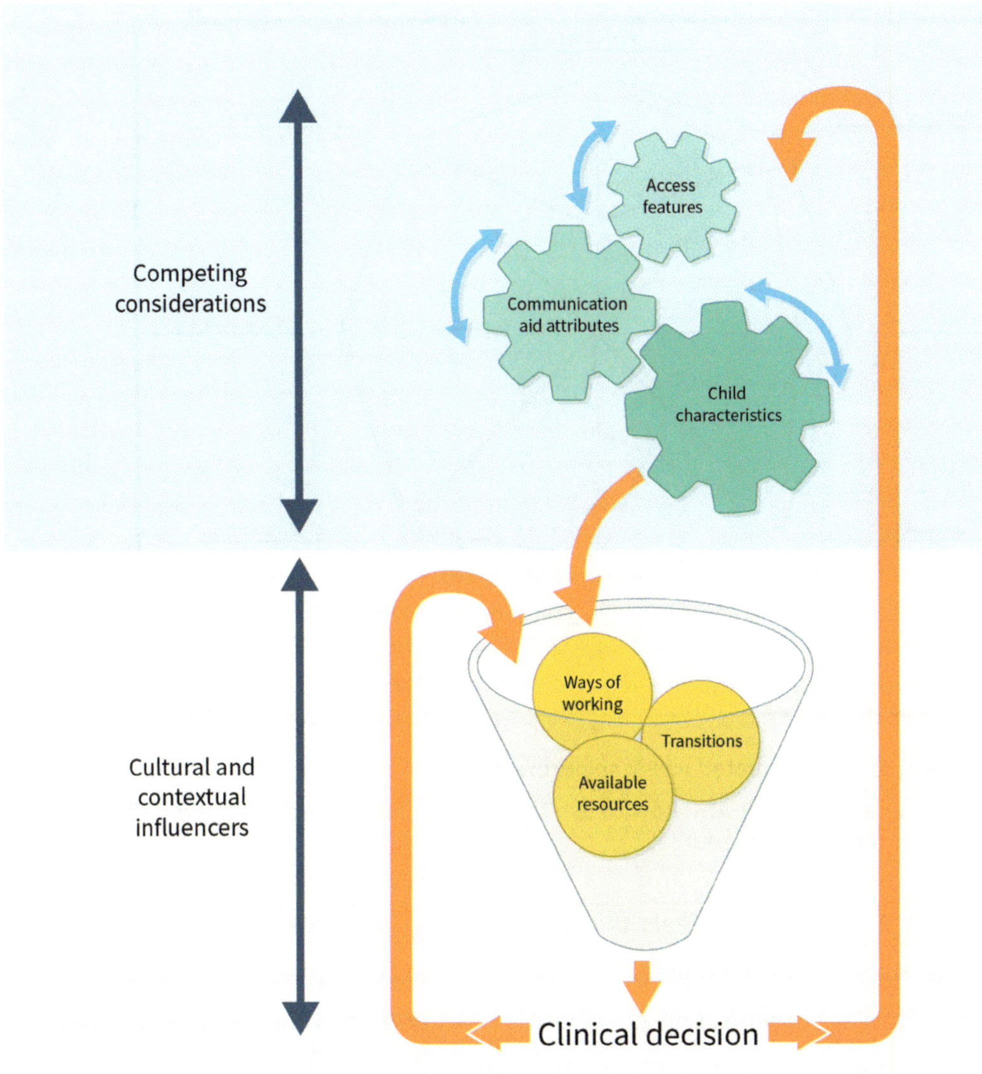

Figure 2.1 The I-ASC Explanatory Model of clinical decision making

Source: reproduced with permission of Janice Murray (first published in Lynch et al., 2019 and Murray et al., 2019, companion papers).

It is also important to consider that each competing considerations is not just competing for priority against the others, but there may be variance in the priorities of the individuals involved in the decision-making process. A more straightforward AAC assessment might be one where each person agrees on the priorities, however this is rarely the case. For example, the education practitioners might feel durability and battery life are the most important features (**hardware** reliability), the speech and language therapist might feel that software vocabulary takes priority and the child may be most concerned about what the communication aid looks like. This is demonstrated in Figure 2.2. The completed spidergram in Figure 2.2. is a resource from the I-ASC website which allows those involved in AAC decision making to compare their priorities and discuss any variance. Figure 2.2

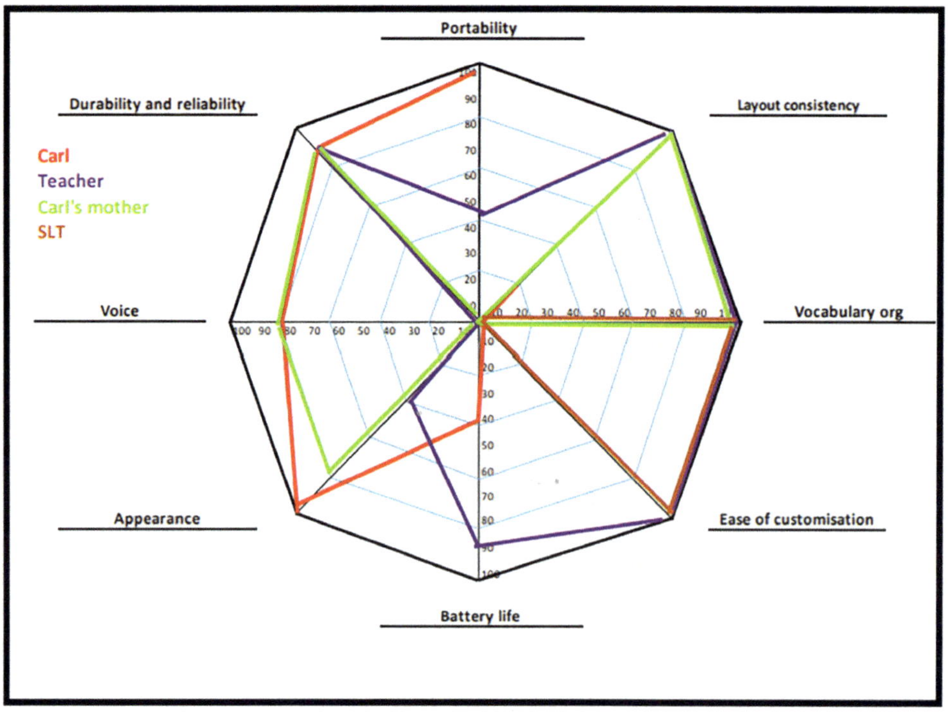

Figure 2.2 Example of a completed I-ASC spidergram

Source: Murray et al. (2020). 'I-ASC how to use the spidergram resource' retrieved 17 May 2023, from https://iasc.mmu.ac.uk/resources/.

shows how the AAC user, Carl, feels that portability, appearance, ease of customisation and the vocabulary organisation are priorities. Carl's teacher agrees that ease of customisation and vocabulary organisation are priorities, but also feels the layout consistency is important. Carl however has rated this as not important to him at all.

The lower half of the I-ASC Explanatory Model of AAC decision making (see Figure 2.1) shows the cultural and contextual influencers which will also affect the decisions which are made. Existing ways of working, the available resources and potential or known transitions in the child's life will interplay with the competing considerations to influence the overall choice of communication aid. The elements from each of the three cultural and contextual influencers can be found here: https://iasc.mmu.ac.uk/wp-content/uploads/2019/05/I-ASC-Cultural-and-contextual-influencers-descriptors.pdf.

Further resources produced as an outcome of the I-ASC study are available at https://iasc.mmu.ac.uk/resources/. These are free to download and will help practitioners at all stages of the communication aid assessment.

For an example of the resources being used with a child, see Lynch and Murray (2023).

What are the decisions that need to be made?

Choosing AAC is rarely an easy decision or a linear path. What is the process that leads us to choose a voice output communication aid for one person and a graphic symbol book for another? Sometimes, we might decide not to use a paper-based book and first try a tablet computer with an app. Other times we might feel sure that paper-based AAC is the right choice and avoid apps altogether. Often, we are left feeling usure where to start at all.

When choosing AAC for someone, asking ourselves the following questions can be helpful:

- What AAC has been tried or used before and what was the outcome?
- What AAC will we trial now?
- How will we decide that we've found the right type of AAC, or that it's time to try something else?

Judge et al. (2023) state: "it is recognised that this decision-making is challenging and inconsistent and that little is known about how practitioners make decisions in practice" (p. 911). The decision-making process has become more complex with the increased availability of tablet computers and AAC apps and fast pace of changes in technology (Light et al., 2019, and Lund et al., 2017, cited in Judge et al., 2023). Decisions are heavily influenced by the child's environment, are based on the **vocabulary package** which the people supporting the AAC user are familiar with, and often made in the absence of empirical evidence.

Judge et al. (2023) carried out interviews and focus groups with people involved in choosing powered communication aids for children and young people. The aim of their study was to understand how communication aid attributes were described by those making decisions and how these attributes were described as impacting on AAC use. They found that decision-makers used a variety of words to describe communication aid attributes, which were sometimes used interchangeably, such as "the name of an AAC software was used to describe a vocabulary package, or an AAC device name was used to describe a vocabulary package" (p. 917). The language used to describe communication aid attributes does not echo the language used in the literature.

Being able to describe the attributes of communication aids can help us to:

1. Identify different area for assessment.
2. Break down decisions so that the overall process is less overwhelming.
3. Troubleshoot by identifying specific things that might not be working for the AAC user.

Box 2.1 offers some definitions of attributes of communication aids.

BOX 2.1 COMMUNICATION AID ATTRIBUTES

Hardware: The physical equipment containing the language, such as the communication book, E-Tran frame, or tablet computer. The term "device" will often be used, especially when referring to powered communication aids.

Access method: The way in which a person makes a selection on their communication aid. For example, using their eyes, their hands or a switch (see Chapter 5).

Software: The computer software used to create the vocabulary. This might be the software used to design and print the graphic symbol board, or the software which offers a choice of graphic symbols or alphabet-based vocabulary packages on a powered communication aid.

Representation method: Communication aids might represent language using letters, written words, photographs or graphic symbols. The term "graphic symbol" is used rather than just "symbol" because spoken and written words are also symbolic.

Organisational method or vocabulary: The way the graphic symbols, words or letters are organised on the communication aid. This might refer to the way the letters are organised on an alphabet chart (e.g., QWERTY or alphabetically), or a commercially produced product. For communication aids using software (either the print out or displayed on a screen), this is often referred to as the "vocabulary package" (see Chapter 5).

Examples of the attributes of four communication aids are given in table 2.1. as a means of further explaining the different attributes.

Table 2.1 Examples of the attributes of four communication aids

	1	*2*	*3*	*4*
Hardware	Accent 1000 communication aid	Paper book	Paper chart	iPad
Access method	Head mouse	Partner assisted scanning	Direct access (touch)	Switch scanning
Software	Nu Voice	Boardmaker	MS word	Grid for iPad
Representation method	Graphic symbols (PRC)	Graphic symbols (PCS)	Letters	Whole words and phrases
Organisation method or vocabulary package	Unity (84 sequenced)	PODD©	QWERTY	Alpha Core

Breaking down the attributes of a communication aid can help clarify the decisions that need to be made when choosing which to try. As one decision is made, the choices available for the remaining components are likely to narrow (Webb et al., 2019).

Not all components can be used interchangeably and this may greatly restrict the options available. For example, if a person needs to access a communication aid using an eye tracker, they might trial a range of eye trackers and settle on one that works best. This eye tracker might only be compatible with one type of software, that perhaps is available only on hardware that comes in two different sizes, and has the option of five graphic symbol vocabularies. The resulting choice of graphic symbol vocabulary is therefore a direct result of the decision around the access method. For someone who isn't as restricted by their access method, such as someone using their hand to touch the screen, their choice of graphic symbol vocabularies will be much wider. The decision-making process for this individual might start with the graphic symbol package and then the software, before considering the hardware. Webb et al. (2019) describe how decision making often involves "trade-offs" (p. 2), where one attribute takes priority over another and influences product choice. Hafsa's story in Box 2.2 gives a real-life example of how a communication aid was chosen.

BOX 2.2 HAFSA'S STORY

Hafsa is 13 years old and has quadriplegic cerebral palsy, profound visual impairment and a learning disability. She is a wheelchair user. She has moderate control of her arms and hands and can use a touch screen on a tablet computer fairly well.

Hafsa currently uses a SuperTalker communication aid, which she accesses with her right hand. The SuperTalker is a battery-operated powered communication aid which adults record messages onto using their voice. Hafsa is usually given a choice of two messages on the SuperTalker, such as "more" and "stop".

Hafsa also uses a partner assisted auditory scanning book. Her communication partner begins by reading out four topic choices including "I want to do something" and "help me". Hafsa can indicate her choice by raising her right arm and vocalising. The communication partner will then read out further choices such as "sing a song", "iPad" and "read a story".

Hafsa's parents feel that she needs to be able to communicate more things than her current AAC allows. They have noticed her responses to conversation, such as laughing or becoming excited, which suggest she understands more language than she is able to express currently.

Following an assessment by her Speech and Language Therapist, the attributes required in a communication aid for Hafsa are described in Table 2.2. The requirement that the communication to speak aloud the selections as she touches the screen (known as **auditory phishing**) and a **pragmatically organised vocabulary** (see Chapter 5) meant that there was only one communication aid available to choose. This example shows how the required attributes will often restrict the range of options that decision-makers have available to choose from.

Table 2.2 An example of the attributes required in for a communication aid

Attribute	*What Hafsa needs*	*Options*
Hardware	About 10 inches and will sit flat onthe tray of her wheelchair. Has environmental control functions.	There are a range of tablets available that meet Hafsa's needs. An iPad wouldn't be ideal because she needs environmental control functions.
Access method	Touch access using her hands. Has auditory highlighting or phishing to speak out the choices asshe touches them. Has a keyguard overlay fitted to help her locate the words.	There are only two software that have the auditory phishing function.
Software	No restrictions other than being easy for adults around her to use.	Most of the software available would be suitable.
Representation method	No restrictions (as she can't see the screen).	Many options.
Organisation method or vocabulary package	Uses pragmatic organisation method she is familiar with from using her partner assisted auditory scanning book.	There is a small range of software that offer a pragmatically organised vocabulary package, only one will allow the use of auditory phishing.

Who is making the decisions?

The key roles involved in an AAC assessments are as follows:

The person

The opinions of the person who will be using AAC should be at the centre of every decision.

The family of the person

Those close to the AAC user, such as parents, carers, children, spouses or partners will be able to provide an insight into their needs and aspirations, often acting as an advocate for the person during the assessment.

Speech and language therapist (SLT)

SLTs will play a fundamental role in assessing the person's speech, language and communication skills which will influence the choice of representation method, organisational method and vocabulary package.

Occupational therapist (OT)

OTs will support the assessment for the AAC access method and mounting equipment and may also play a role with sensory and cognition assessments.

Educational practitioners

Teachers and teaching assistants will support the assessment by providing information about the young person's communication, physical, cognitive and literacy skills. They will also be able to provide information about the school environment and any factors regarding this which might influence choices regarding AAC.

Other practitioners

Depending on where the person lives and their healthcare needs, there may be other practitioners such as nurses, key workers, support workers, doctors and Physiotherapists who may have an influence on AAC choices.

While the above definitions define the practitioner and family member roles, the I-ASC study (Murray et al., 2019) highlights how we might view roles in terms of the expectations placed on each person in the decision-making process. These include titles such as the "receiver of information" and "co-ordinator". See the resource "choosing roles in AAC decision making" found here: https://iasc.mmu.ac.uk/wp-content/uploads/2019/04/I-ASC-Choosing-roles-in-AAC-decision-making-and-implementation.pdf

Open AAC

The **OpenAAC** initiative aims to encourage AAC product developers to provide AAC tools which are open-licensed, allowing AAC users to "mix and match" the components of their AAC with fewer restrictions or trade-offs.

The OpenAAC initiative have identified nine key elements which are often restricted in some way:

- **Systems:** AAC hardware or software might be subject to "vendor lock-in".
- **Symbols:** Practitioners might not be able to use the symbols from an AAC system to create other resources.
- **Exports:** AAC software might prevent the user from sharing their vocabulary package to other communication aids if they choose to use something else.
- **Vocabularies:** AAC users might be restricted to a certain communication aid because of the vocabulary package they wish to use.
- **Lessons:** There is often a charge for tools or resources which support AAC learning.
- **Assessments:** AAC assessment resources are often costly and not easily accessible.
- **Research:** Data about how people use AAC is often not freely available. This information can help communication aid manufacturers to design new systems if it were freely available.
- **Integrations:** Websites and other software might not be compatible with a person's powered communication aid.
- **Voices:** Some voices are costly and AAC users might be forced to choose a voice they don't like if they can't afford the one they want.

For further information on the OpenAAC initiative, visit www.openaac.org/

Ways of gathering information

Asking people

Information gathering should always begin by talking to the people that know the person well, and talking to the person themselves, which might require the use of tools such as Talking Mats (see Chapter 4). The two assessment forms provided in this chapter will help guide the questions which need to be asked.

It is also helpful to ask about the people that the person interacts with during their daily life. The Social Networks inventory (Blackstone and Hunt-Berg, 2003) provides an overview of all the people a person communicates with and supports practitioners to determine appropriate communication strategies.

Observing

Meeting the person and observing their communication skills in a familiar setting will always be a valuable way to gather information about them. If they split their time between two or more settings, such as a day centre and family home, then it will be beneficial to observe them in each place. Observing their interactions with a range of people can also be useful. An observation checklist has been provided in this chapter to support information gathering. Other observation checklists are available online. A blog post titled "AAC assessment forms" from Carole Zangari (2014) lists a range of assessment forms and checklists which practitioners may wish to consider.

Activities

Sometimes it will be helpful to investigate specific skills that cannot easily be determined by observing the person during their daily activities. This might include their level of understanding of spoken language, their understanding of graphic symbols or literacy skills.

Formal language assessments can be helpful in some cases, providing the person is able to access them. Many receptive language assessments require the person to either manipulate objects or point to pictures. For lots of AAC users, doing either or both of these things can be challenging which might mean they are unable to complete form language assessments. Practitioners should consider how assessments might be adapted to allow a person with motor impairments to access them.

In many cases where pictures are used, instead of pointing the person could use partner assisted scanning, where the communication partner points to the pictures in turn and waits for confirmation from the person (see Chapter 6 for more information).

Where objects are used, it might be possible to use photographs or symbols to offer an alternative way to access the assessment items. For example, if you wanted to ask the person to "put the teddy under the chair" you could photograph the teddy and chair in four different positions and ask the person to point to "which photo shows teddy under the chair?"

The Computer Based Accessible Receptive Language Assessment (CARLA) supports receptive language assessment via alternative access methods using a computer.

https://mindexpress.jabbla.com/en/download/carla/

It is important that when undertaking an assessment with someone using alternative access methods such as eye pointing or scanning that you are confident, they can use this access method. Asking someone to participate in an assessment without prior experience of the access method would mean the results would be unreliable. There are some assessments which are designed to look at skills specific to AAC.

The Frenchay screening tool for AAC

www.nbt.nhs.uk/bristol-centre-enablement/services-at-centre/aac-west-service/aac-west-products

This assessment provided a range of assessment categories including:

- Physical access
- Visual acuity
- Visual processing
- Visual contrast sensitivity
- Identifying different types of symbols
- Categorisation
- Word-picture matching
- Reading and spelling (with and without symbol support)

Test of aided communication (TASP)

https://goboardmaker.com/products/tasp

This assessment supports practitioners to understand a person's understanding and use of graphic symbols, with subtests for:

- Symbol size and number
- Grammatical encoding
- Categorisation
- Syntactic performance

It will also design communication board layouts and suggest goals for the person.

AAC assessment observation checklist

Name		Date	
Setting		Activity	
People present			
Person's mood and presentation (e.g., tired, excited, distressed, tearful, happy)			
Motor and sensory skills			
Multimodal communication skills (describe if and how it was used and how successful it was)			
Eye pointing			
Gestures			
Manual signing			
Vocalisations			
Spoken words			
Paper/printed AAC			
Powered AAC			

Who did they interact with?
Reasons for communicating (e.g. giving information, self-regulation, requesting)
Opportunities for communicating
Communication breakdowns (describe the interaction and when the breakdown occurred)
Communication partner skills (what did they do to support the person? What might they have done to help?)
Further observations or comments

How do we know when we've found the right AAC?

Decision making can often focus on what AAC to choose, but there is often less guidance available on how to tell when the AAC chosen is working well and worth continuing with, or when to stop and try something else. In an ideal world, everyone would hope that the person quickly begins to use the AAC and demonstrates that they see its value. The reality is that we may not see this for many weeks or months. Sometimes this perceived lack of progress can be disheartening for the people supporting the person, who might be expecting them to start communicating using the AAC relatively quickly.

Choosing how long to trial a communication aid for can be a difficult decision. Factors which might impact the length of an AAC trial might include:

- Periods of illness, for the person or those supporting them.
- Planned or unplanned hospital admissions.
- Life events, such as the birth or a sibling or death of a loved one.
- Transitions between settings, such as a house move or change of school, or a move between hospital care and a care home.
- Loss of one or more of the team supporting the AAC user, such as a key worker resigning from their role.
- Holidays.
- Competing therapy or rehabilitation programmes which take priority, such as the need for a period of intense physiotherapy.
- Sleep difficulties.

Any of these reasons may extend the length of the AAC trial considerably, or lead to the trial being delayed or paused for a period. It is important to take these factors into account when evaluating a person's experience of using AAC.

AAC trial goals

It is important to begin any AAC trials by discussion expectations and defining goals for the assessment. Where funding routes exist, it is easy to be led down the path of setting goals to meet the funding criteria, which should never be the aim. Trialling AAC should also not focus on developing competencies with the communication aid, as this will take many months or years.

AAC trials are for:

- Checking that the communication aid chosen meets the person's needs in terms of reliability, design and durability.
- Making sure the person can use the access method with the communication aid.
- Ensuring people around the person are able to support them to use the communication aid.
- Making sure that the person is motivated to use the communication aid.

AAC trials are not for:

- Proving that someone meets criteria for funding.
- Demonstrating that someone can communicate "competently" (see Chapter 7 for further discussion on this idea).

Some suggested goals are given here:

- For *(insert name)* to show repeated motivation to use the communication aid.
- For *(insert name)* to be able to successfully and consistently use the chosen access method.

It is important to record progress during trials of AAC. This can help everyone share successes and challenges which will help with future planning. A template for a progress record form has been provided.

What to do when there is difference in opinion

Unfortunately, there may be times where people involved in choosing AAC do not agree. This may be relating to the competing consideration as detailed in the I-ASC Explanatory Model of AAC decision making (see Figure 2.1).

First, it's important to listen to everyone's views and give them the opportunity to share their opinions. Ultimately, the decision is likely to be made by the person who has access to or responsibility for allocating the funding. This can mean that this person might be seen as the "gatekeeper" and having more power than others.

Sometimes, the decision not to provide a certain type of AAC may be made. Family members might be disappointed and seek alternative sources of funding, such as charity or self-funding. This can pose a particular conflict if the family then ask the AAC user's daytime setting (such as school, college or day centre) to implement their preferred AAC. Conflict may also arise when families choose to follow a support programme or method which goes against the values or professional guidelines of practitioners or the setting. On these occasions, it is important to:

- Offer everyone the opportunity to voice their opinions about what is right for the person.
- Provide the person with the opportunity to contribute to the discussions as much as possible.

- Support any decisions with reasoning, which might include evidence, good practice guidelines or position statements.
- Acknowledge the differences in opinion and understand the reasons for this.

Additionally, it may be appropriate to offer a second opinion or assessment. A compromise may be able to be reached, as sometimes it might be possible and appropriate to use two types of AAC in parallel, for example agreeing to use both the communication aid with the eye tracker and a partner assisted scanning symbol chart, at different points throughout the day.

If it has been decided that a particular type of AAC will not be provided, offering clear goals to work towards and a time frame for review can be helpful, for example, "Now isn't the right time, but we can work on developing X skills. When he/she/they have chieved X we can think again about trying this again."

Summary

Choosing AAC for someone is often a complex process and always dependent on a range of factors. It is also not just about the skills and needs of the person themselves, but also influenced by their environment, the people supporting them and existing ways of working. Theoretical models can help us to understand the competing considerations and contextual influencers.

Assessment is a process of gathering information, across a range of contexts and via different methods. Traditional language assessments may not suit this population and assessments may need to be adapted to meet a person's access needs. Informal observations and talking to the people that know the person well are always valuable assessment tools.

When trialling AAC, it's important to have clear goals for the trial period and understand what success will look like within a given time frame. Factors such as health, available support and holiday periods may impact on how long AAC needs to be trialled. Communication is key and practitioners should endeavour to include everyone in the decision-making process. Sometimes, not everyone will agree with decisions that are made and it's important to have strategies to deal with any conflict.

AAC trial record form

Date	*Activity*	*People*	*Example of AAC use*	*Any challenges*	*Additional comments*
Example *16/06/25*	*Example* *Breakfast time*	*Example* *Mum, Jack, Sally*	*Example* *Jack found the word toast and answer my question*	*Example* *The page closed after he pressed toast but Jack wanted to say more and got annoyed*	*Sally likes helping Jack find the words*

References

Bailey, R. W. (1996). *Human performance Engineering: Designing High Quality, Professional User Interfaces for Computer Products, Applications, and Systems* (3rd ed.). Prentice Hall.

Blackstone, S. and Hunt-Berg, M. (2003). *Social Networks: A communication Inventory for the Individuals with Complex Communication Needs and Their Communication Partners*. Attainment Company.

Judge, S., Murray, J., Lynch, Y., Meredith, S., Moulam, L., Randall, N., Whittle, H. and Goldbart, J. (2023). Attributes of communication aids as described by those supporting children and young people with AAC. *International Journal of Language & Communication Disorders*, 58, 910–928. https://doi.org/10.1111/1460-6984.12833/.

Light, J., McNaughton, D., Beukelman, D., Fager, S.K., Fried-Oken, M., Jakobs, T., et al. (2019). Challenges and opportunities in augmentative and alternative communication: research and technology development to enhance communication and participation for individuals with complex communication needs. *Augmentative and Alternative Communication*, 35(1), 1–12. https://doi.org/10. 1080/07434618.2018.1556732.

Lund, S.K., Quach, W., Weissling, K., McKelvey, M. & Dietz, A. (2017). Assessment with children who need augmentative and alternative communication (AAC): clinical decisions of AAC specialists. *Language, Speech, and Hearing Services in Schools*, 48(1), 56–68. https://doi.org/10.1044/2016_LSHSS-15-0086

Lynch, Y. and Murray, J. (2023). The I-ASC Explanatory Model as a support for AAC assessment planning: A case report. In M. M. Smith (ed.) (2023) *Clinical Cases in Augmentative and Alternative Communication* (1st ed.). Routledge. https://doi.org/10.4324/9781003106739/.

Lynch, Y., Murray, J., Moulam, L., Meredith, S., Goldbart, J., Smith, M., Batorowicz, B., Randall, N. Judge, S. (2019). Decision making in communication aid recommendations in the UK: Cultural and contextual influencers. *Augmentative and Alternative Communication*. 35(3): 180-192. http://doi: 10.1080/07434618.2019.1599066.

Murray, J., Lynch, Y., Meredith, S., Moulam, L., Goldbart, J., Smith, M., Randall, N. and Judge, S. (2019). Professionals' decision making in recommending communication aids in the UK: Competing considerations. *Augmentative and Alternative Communication*, 35(3): 167–179. DOI: 10.1080/07434618.2019.1597384.

Murray, J., Lynch, Y., Goldbart, J., Moulam, L., Judge, S., Webb, E., Jayes, M., Meredith, D., Whittle, H., Randall, N., Meads, D. and Hess, S. (2020). The decision-making process in recommending electronic communication aids for children and young people who are non-speaking: the I-ASC mixed-methods study. *Health Serv Deliv Res*, 8(45). www.journalslibrary.nihr.ac.uk/hsdr/hsdr08450/#/abstract.

Scherer, M. J. (2005). *Living in the State of Stuck: How Assistive Technology Impacts the Lives of People with Disabilities* (4th ed.). Brookline Books.

Scherer, M. J. and Federici, S. (2015). Why people use and don't use technologies: Introduction to the special issue on assistive technologies for cognition/cognitive support technologies, *NeuroRehabilitation*, 37, 315–319. IOS Press, DOI: 10.3233/NRE-151264.

Webb, E. J. D., Lynch, Y., Meads, D., Judge, S., Randall, N., Goldbart, J., Meredith, S., Moulam, L., Hess, S. and Murray, J. (2019). Finding the best fit: Examining the decision-making of augmentative and alternative communication professionals in the UK using a discrete choice experiment, *BMJ Open*, 9: e030274. https://doi.org/10.1136/bmjopen-2019-030274.

Williams, M. B., Krezman, C. and McNaughton, D. (2008). "Reach for the Stars": Five principles for the next 25 years of AAC. *Augmentative Alternative Communication*, 24, 194-206. https://doi.org/10.1080/08990220802387851.

Zangari, C. (2014, 30 October). AAC assessment forms, *Practical AAC blog*. https://praacticalaac.org/praactical/aac-assessment-forms/.

3

WHAT MAKES A GOOD AAC SERVICE?

Helen Robinson

DOI: 10.4324/9781003412311-4

What does "good" look like?

The term "AAC service" might be used to describe an individual or team that provides support for AAC users. The term *service* can be problematic, as it alludes to a provider and consumer model, the practitioner(s) being the provider(s) and the AAC user being the consumer or customer. "AAC provision" and "AAC intervention" are also terms which might not be liked or understood by AAC users. The term "communication supports" might be preferable (Zisk and Konyn, 2022). While acknowledging that the term AAC service may be disliked or not understood, it is also important to note its relevance when discussing the pathways of support available for people. Services might be privately funded, not-for-profit charities or commissioned by health or education providers. Services might be one person, a global company employing hundreds of people or something in between. Often services work together or alongside each other to support AAC users.

There is much documentation available to practitioners regarding what a good AAC service might look like. This is often linked to local and national policy. Region- and country-specific policies or pathways are not explained here, but instead the aim is to offer guidance as to what a "good" experience of an AAC service might look like for someone who uses it (a service user) and the fundamentals required of a service to be able to offer this.

The broad aim of an AAC service is to provide alternative and augmentative communication methods to those who would benefit from them, so that they can communicate to their full potential. The service must also meet the changing needs of a person, for as long as they need AAC. Often, several teams or services might be involved in AAC assessment and support. Transition between services should be seamless, without gaps in care for the person and unnecessary worry about which service they qualify for and how to access the right practitioners or funding streams. Multiple funding streams are common across AAC services and ideally the service user shouldn't need to be concerned about this. Each stage of the person's care should flow seamlessly without the person having to navigate between and understand varying referral criteria and care pathways.

Service standards

The "Augmentative and Alternative (AAC) Service Standards" document from Communication Matters (2012) sets out a number of Quality Statements for AAC Services and provides the reader with key policy papers and good practice documents. These service standards serve as a useful audit tool for existing AAC services and a helpful baseline for new services and are reproduced here with permission from Communication Matters. For the full document please visit: www.communicationmatters.org.uk/resources/publications/.

Quality standard for AAC services

The quality statements are written from the perspective of the AAC speaker and should be taken to mean the individual themselves and/or their family or support worker who is authorised to make a decision with and on behalf of that individual if they are a child or someone without the ability to make decisions independently.

- I can expect to have the right to equal access to an AAC service regardless of:
  - Age or time of onset of impairment
  - Severity of impairment
  - Geographical location
  - Economic status
  - Linguistic or cultural background
- I can expect to be involved in an assessment process that is demonstrably impartial, independent and objective.
- I can expect to receive a high-quality, fair and personal service from an AAC service.
- I can expect the practitioners working with me to share information, knowledge and skills.
- I can expect the practitioners working with me to communicate effectively with each other for my best interests.
- I can expect all members of the AAC service to have the required skills, knowledge and competencies.
- I can expect my knowledge, skills and experience to be valued and acknowledged.
- I can expect to be involved as an active participant throughout the whole decision-making process.
- I can expect that, if my needs for AAC cannot be addressed by my current team, a referral will be made to a team with the appropriate knowledge, skills and experience.
- I can expect my local SLT/ AAC team, and the AAC specialist service to have a care pathway that describes their part in the management of my AAC needs.
- I can expect to be informed where to go for a second opinion if the AAC service does not meet my needs.

Reproduced with permission from: Quality Standard for AAC Services (2011). Communication Matters (p. 6). These quality standards are due to be updated imminently and the latest version can be found on the Communication Matters website.

The Royal College of Speech and Language Therapists (RCSLT, 2024) have produced a set of 16 guidelines for supporting AAC users, which cover seven themes of AAC practice, including: AAC user identity, AAC service structures and AAC intervention.

In the United Kingdom the Community Equipment Code of Practice Scheme (CECOPS) aims to raise the standards of assistive technology services. It is an independent not-for-profit certification and standards body which evaluates the commissioning, provision and clinical element of assistive technology services. The CECOPS framework and self-evaluation tool provides services with standards against which they can measure themselves. Services can gain accreditation which lets service users know that they are meeting the recommended standards. See https://www.cecops.org.uk/ for further details.

The AAC care pathway

Care pathways describe the different stages or steps in the support provided to a person.

There is great variability amongst the care pathways for AAC services, regionally, nationally and globally. Each care pathway will be heavily influenced by local and national policy, how services are commissioned and how they link in with other services. If care pathways are made freely available to the public, they can help someone understand what their journey might look like. They serve as a means to ensure everyone within a defined geographical area receives the same standard of support, but should also allow for the circumstances and needs of the individual person.

An example of the different stages of AAC support for a person is given in Figure 3.1. Each element of the care pathway is described along with important considerations and questions to ask.

Identification

Before anyone can access an AAC service, they are often dependent on practitioners being aware of what AAC is and being able to identify that they might benefit from using it, or the person themselves or their family need to know what AAC is in order to know that AAC may be beneficial and seek the required support.

The practitioners in AAC services should continuously seek to raise awareness among the practitioners in other services who have the potential to identify that a person might benefit from AAC and refer into their service. These might be speech and language

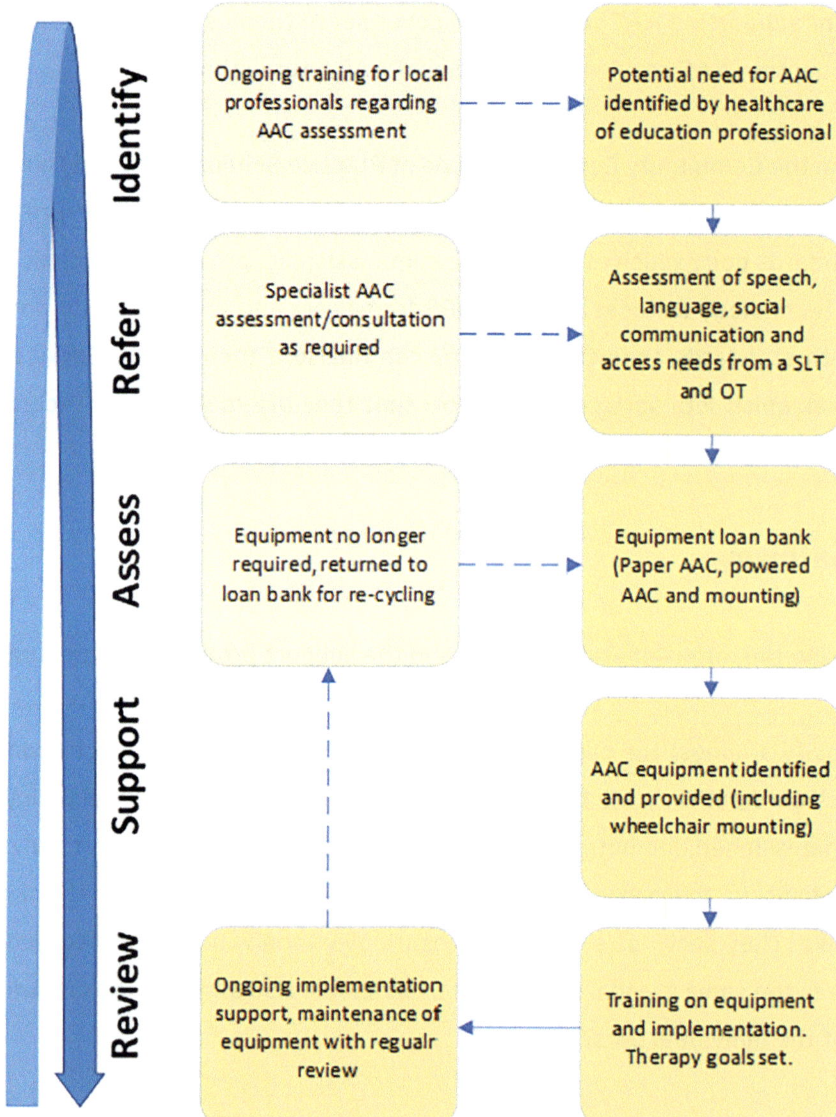

Figure 3.1 A proposed care pathway

Source: AAC in South Yorkshire, Clarke et al. (2022) for The Barnsley Assistive Technology Team (unpublished).

therapists, occupational therapists, teachers and medical practitioners such as doctors and consultants.

As well as considering those people who are most likely to refer to the AAC service, thought must be given to the people or groups that might be involved with a person before they have accessed these services. For example, personal assistants, carers, charity workers, support workers, doctors and volunteers. This might be referred to as developing awareness of AAC at a universal level. Awareness raising might take the form of a training programme, or educational materials such as service information leaflets, posters or a web page.

BOX 3.1 THOUGHTS ON THE CHALLENGES OF DEVELOPING A CARE PATHWAY BY EMILY SINGLETON, SPEECH AND LANGUAGE THERAPIST

I have recently updated the care pathway for our service. The main challenges have been around supporting less confident staff to initially see AAC as something to consider, and secondly to trial systems.

One challenge for those in AAC services is understanding the needs of the local population and identifying the services and practitioners that serve it. Mapping the services across the footprint of the AAC service is essential. Those practitioners in individual services then have an onward responsibility to raise awareness within the communities they support.

Consideration must also be given to healthcare inequalities. The National Health Service (NHS) in the United Kingdom describes these as "unfair and avoidable differences in health across the population, and between different groups within society. These include how long people are likely to live, the health conditions they may experience and the care that is available to them" (NHS England, 2023).

Factors such as the place someone is born, grows up, lives and works can impact their health. Living in an area of high deprivation, belonging to Black, Asian and Minority Ethnic (BAME) communities or being homeless make someone at risk of experiencing healthcare inequalities. Other groups at risk include people with a learning disability, autistic people and people with mental health needs. Factors such as access to transport, literacy skills, previous negative experiences of healthcare services, lack of affordable childcare may all be reasons why a person finds it harder to access an AAC assessment.

The NHS uses the term "Inclusion health groups" to describe people who may be socially excluded and therefore at greater risk of experiencing healthcare inequalities. This includes Gypsy, Roma and Traveller communities, vulnerable migrants, people with drug and alcohol dependence, people in contact with the justice system and people who experience homelessness.

Referral

Practitioners working in AAC services must ensure that other practitioners, or the public (if self-referral is permitted), know how to make a referral to their service. Information about the AAC service and its care pathway should be easily accessible, for example, via the team's website and/or leaflets or posters. Criteria for accessing the service should be freely available. The referral form, email address or the telephone number should be easy to find. Easy read versions of all information should be available.

Making a referral isn't simply a case of knowing where to find the form, it is also about having the necessary skills to gather the information required and provide this to the AAC service. AAC services have a responsibility to help referrers understand what information they need to gather, why it is needed and how to get it. Incomplete or poor-quality referrals are likely to lead to a delay in a person accessing an AAC service. Training on how to complete a good quality referral may be part of general awareness-raising training or information in a leaflet or on a website. A suggested referral form is included here.

AAC assessment referral form

Full name				
Preferred first name				
Gender	male	Female	Non-binary	Other:
Pronouns	He/him/his	She/her/hers	They/them/theirs	Other:
Date of birth				
NHS number of Reference number				
Preferred contact method (email, telephone, text message, letter)				
Home address				
Next of kin name and relation				
Next of kin contact information				
Daytime address (if different to home address)				
Details of key contact person at daytime address				

<table>
<tr>
<td rowspan="4">Home language(s)

Tick ALL languages the child HEARS or SPEAKS

Languages listed are commonly encountered in the UK. This is not an exhaustive list.

Please adapt to your catchment/case load</td>
<td>Pakistani-heritage languages:
□ Mirpuri
□ Punjabi
□ Urdu</td>
<td>Asian & African-heritage languages
□ Arabic
□ Turkish
□ Persian/Farsi
□ Somali
□ Tagalog/Filipino</td>
</tr>
<tr>
<td>Bangladeshi-heritage languages:
□ Sylheti
□ Standard Bangla</td>
<td rowspan="3">European-heritage languages:
□ English
□ French
□ German
□ Italian
□ Lithuanian
□ Polish
□ Portuguese
□ Romanian
□ Spanish
□ Other:</td>
</tr>
<tr>
<td>Indian-heritage languages:
□ Guajarati
□ Tamil</td>
</tr>
<tr>
<td>Chinese-heritage languages:
□ Putonghua
□ Cantonese</td>
</tr>
<tr>
<td>Is an interpreter helpful for the assessment of the person, informed consent, and/or discussion with the parent(s)/carer?</td>
<td colspan="2"></td>
</tr>
<tr>
<td>Heritage/Ethnicity</td>
<td colspan="2"></td>
</tr>
<tr>
<td>Has this person or their next of kin consented to this referral?</td>
<td colspan="2"></td>
</tr>
<tr>
<td>Other practitioners involved</td>
<td colspan="2"></td>
</tr>
<tr>
<td>Does the person have a diagnosis?
If so, please list the diagnosis/diagnoses and when this was given</td>
<td colspan="2"></td>
</tr>
<tr>
<td>If the person has a degenerative condition, please describe the rate of the progression</td>
<td colspan="2"></td>
</tr>
</table>

Describe how communication attempts might be unsuccessful for this person. What are they wanting to communicate but can't?	
Describe this person's history of AAC use Include what has been tried, what has not worked well and what has been successful.	
What are the reasons for making this referral? Consider what you as the referrer might hope to gain, and what the person being referred might hope to gain from this assessment.	
Name	
Role	
Contact details	
Date of referral	
Adapted from a speech and language therapy referral from by Sean Pert (2023). Working with Children Experiencing Speech and Language Disorders in a Bilingual Context: A Home Language Approach (pp. 49–50). With permission from Routledge.	

Assessment

An AAC service should include a range of practitioners, including but not limited to, speech and language therapists, occupational therapists, administrative assistants, healthcare scientists, teachers, technologists and technicians. There are competency tools available to support the developing knowledge and skills of each practitioner, including:

- The Informing and Profiling Augmentative and Alternative Communication (AAC) Knowledge and Skills (IP**AAC**KS) was developed for NHS Education for Scotland, building on previous documents, including the AAC Competencies Project for the charity Communication Matters. The aim of the IPAACKs document is to ensure practitioners supporting AAC users have the required knowledge, skills and values to improve the experiences, opportunities and quality of life of AAC users (NHS Education for Scotland, 2014). It does this by providing a framework for practitioners to identify the necessary skills required for their role, and then map their current competencies onto. It is freely downloadable from: www.aacscotland.org.uk/files/cm/files/ipaacks.pdf.

- The Barnsley Assistive Technology Team (2021) have produced a competency framework for the role of Assistive Technology Specialist, which can be freely downloaded from their website. It covers the following areas of competency:
    - Service delivery and commissioning
    - Assistive Technology Equipment and Techniques
    - Equipment management
    - The person
    - Assessment, decision making and goal setting
    - Training
    - Research

Assessments need to be accessible for each service user. If possible, people should be given choice of where their assessment takes place and who attends. McNaughton et al. (2018) surveyed 21 people and concluded that the following three principles are key to AAC assessment and intervention:

- appropriate staging of the timing of assessment and intervention activities
- inclusion of communication partners
- the use of multiple modalities and strategies as communication supports

Details of a high-quality AAC assessment are given in Chapters 4 and 5. Practitioners will need access to equipment to be able to carry out a complete assessment (an equipment loan bank). A checklist is provided for services to consider the equipment they have available to them.

Checklist for equipment loan bank for AAC services

	Equipment	*Sufficient amount? Yes/no*	*Comments*
HARDWARE AND SOFTWARE	Software to allow the production of paper-based AAC resources (may be ongoing subscriptions).		
	Communication aid software for preparing and editing AAC vocabularies.		
	AAC apps		
	Eye pointing communication aides e.g., Eye link board or E-Tran frame.		
	Alphabet based powered communication aids		
	Powered communication aids with graphic symbols		
	Recorded message communication aids.		
ACCESS METHODS	Basic switches e.g., buddy button		
	Specialised switches e.g., string switch, chin switch, wobble switch.		
	Eye trackers		
	Head mouse		
	Key guards		
	Adapted mice		
	Alternative keyboards		
	Alternative styluses		
MOUNTS	Table top mounts		
	Wheelchair mounts		
	Floor stands		
	Mounting for switches		
FACILITIES	Equipment to facilitate voice banking – laptop, software and high-quality microphone.		
	Paper and printing facilities to produce paper communication aids. Matt, waterproof, non-tearing paper is preferred.		

AAC equipment provision

A service must have skilled practitioners who are able to prepare (set up) the equipment prior to loan. This equipment may need adapting to meet the needs of an individual. This might be the software that requires configuring to meet their sensory needs, or the hardware which requires adapting or even custom manufacture. For example, a custom-made wheelchair mount to hold the communication aid. The communication aid may need integrating with the person's powered wheelchair; this is the process where some powered wheelchairs can be connected, usually via blue tooth, to the communication aid. The wheelchair controls can then also be used to control the communication aid, with the ability to switch between driving the chair and using the communication aid.

Once the appropriate equipment has been identified, there should be funding available to provide this on long-term loan to the person. AAC services should communicate to the service user or their representative the terms of the equipment loan. This should include:

- Who owns the equipment.
- What the expectations are of the AAC user and/or their representative regarding insurance of the equipment and how to look after it.
- What will happen if the equipment is lost, damaged or stolen.
- What the equipment can and cannot be used for. For example, can the user download software onto the communication aid? Are they allowed to add their own apps to the iPad? Are they allowed to use the tablet for purposes other than communicating?
- What will happen if the person breaks the terms of the agreement?

AAC services should keep an accurate record of what equipment has been provided to each person and when it has been returned.

Support

An AAC service must be able to support the person and any equipment provided throughout their lifespan, or until AAC is no longer required. Initially, training must be provided to the person and those supporting them. Further training may be required along the person's AAC journey. Further details on the support required to use AAC are given in Chapter 7.

AAC services must have the ability to maintain and manage the equipment for as long as the communication aid is in use. This includes having the skills to repair the equipment when it breaks, loan temporary equipment while under repair and replace equipment when it is no longer functional. Systems must be in place to ensure the appropriate disposal of faulty equipment.

Equipment management goes beyond fixing and replacing. Powered communication aids will inevitably require software updates and manufacturer recalls. AAC services must have procedures in place so they know where their equipment is, inform the AAC users, rectify the issue and potentially provide a loan communication aid temporarily.

Procedures must be in place to ensure any equipment is clean and minimise the risk of infection. Services should have a designated area for cleaning used equipment, and the resources to do so.

Procedures must be considered for ensuring a person's data is managed. It should be clear who owns and controls any personal data on the communication aid. When equipment is returned to the AAC service, steps must be in place to ensure effective data cleansing.

Review

AAC support for a person is rarely ever linear, and to view it as such is perhaps where services often fail. It is not simply a case of assessing and providing AAC. A person's needs are likely to change over time and an effective AAC service must be able to respond to this.

Whether that's the loss of skills if the person has a degenerative condition, or it could be that the person gains skills, either physically or linguistically. Either way, they will need their AAC to adapt to meet these changes. Sometimes, if the person has a rapidly deteriorating condition, these changes will occur often and the level of support will need to be high. For other people, their abilities may be stable for a number of years and they may need support from a service infrequently.

A person's environment might change, meaning they need a little extra support for a while. AAC users will likely transition across different settings throughout their life, such as one school to another, from children's services into adult services, or between community and acute settings.

The people around the AAC user are also likely to change, often linked to a change in environment, but not always. This might require additional training to be provided.

Even when the person, the environment and the people around them are stable, the AAC itself might break or reach the end of its life, again calling for additional support.

Additional to the needs of the person, it is important to ensure any equipment is reviewed regularly (at least annually) to ensure it is in good, safe, working order. For example, checking for any damage and testing the power supply. Thinking of AAC support as being ongoing, or cyclical, is a good place to start when considering how to develop an effective AAC service.

Checklist to review an AAC care pathway

	Consideration	*Yes*	*No*	*Comments*
IDENTIFICATION	Does your service offer accessible training so that people can identify when a person might benefit from being referred for an AAC assessment?			
	Do you have an understanding of your local population?			
	Has your service mapped the services that might play a role in identifying that a person might benefit from AAC?			
	Have you considered people who might be at increased risk of not being able to access your service due to healthcare inequalities and how you might respond to this risk?			
REFERRAL	Can people easily find information about your service and is this accessible?			
	Does your referral ask the questions that will give you good quality information about the person?			
	Do you have processes in place to manage referrals which do not meet your service's referral criteria?			
	What support/signposting, if any, can you offer to people not meeting criteria for your service?			
ASSESSMENT	How does your service ensure your practitioners are competent to perform their role?			
	What Clinical Supervision processes do you have in place?			
	Is the service user's opinion sought during assessment?			
	Do practitioners have access to the tools they need to carry out a comprehensive assessment?			

	Consideration	Yes	No	Comments
EQUIPMENT PROVISION	Can your service adapt AAC equipment to meet the individual needs of each person?			
	Can your service mount the person's communication aid so they can use it when needed (e.g., wheelchair, bed, armchair, standing frame).			
	Do you communicate the terms of the equipment loan to the person or their representative in an accessible way?			
	Do you have an accurate record of each piece of equipment that has been loaned?			
SUPPORT	Does each person receive training about their AAC equipment?			
	Do the people supporting the AAC user receive the training they need to do this well?			
	Does your service have an adequate supply of equipment to provide people with temporary a loan if theirs breaks?			
	Do AAC users and those who support them know who to contact when something stops working, and how to do this?			
	Are systems in place to protect the personal data of AAC users?			
	Do AAC users know who has responsibility for managing (controlling) their data?			
	Are systems in place to prevent infections when transferring equipment between people?			
REVIEW	Can people come back into the service when their needs change?			
	Can people access further assessment when needed?			
	During times of transition, is additional training available for people who come into the person's life?			
	Are processes in place to review the safe use of any equipment provided?			

How to seek funding for an AAC service

The information provided in this section has been adapted from the website "Local AAC Services Commissioning Toolkit" (14 March 2023). The toolkit was developed jointly by a working party of practitioners working in AAC services across England. The website is a useful resource for practitioners in the UK looking to develop an AAC service, with links to many useful documents and legislation applicable to England. The process of seeking funding for an AAC service is shown in Figure 3.2 and then described in detail.

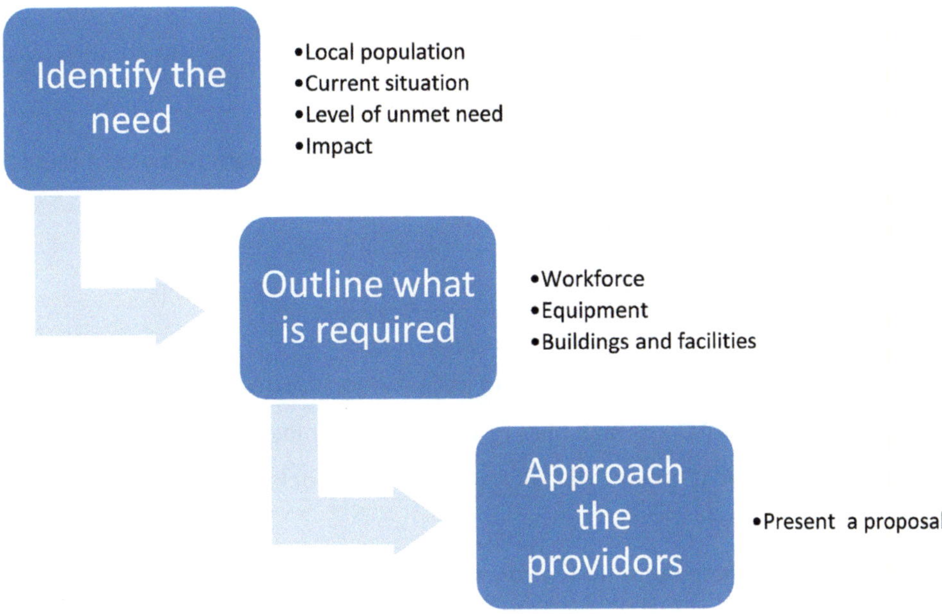

Figure 3.2 The process of seeking funding for an AAC service

Identify the need for a service

When building a case for an AAC service, the first step is to explain why that service is needed. Set the context by explaining what AAC is and who might use it. Consider the local population size and the prevalence of AAC. It is known that 0.6% of the population will require AAC (Blackstone et al., cited in Communication Matters, 2011). Finding out the population of the area the AAC service will serve and multiplying by 0.6, then dividing by 100 will give the number of people requiring AAC for that area.

Explain the current situation; what care pathway is in place? Why isn't this working?

Gather data on the anticipated unmet need of the local population. Using surveys is a useful way to investigate where good practice exists and where the gaps are. Questions to ask might include the following topics:

- Are practitioners able to identify when someone might benefit from AAC?
- Are practitioners skilled in assessing for AAC?
- Do practitioners have access to training and continued practitioner development, including supervision?
- Do practitioners have access to a loan bank of equipment for assessment?
- Is equipment funded when assessment indicates it would be beneficial?
- Are their systems in pace to ensure the appropriate management of AAC equipment?

- Do AAC users have regular reviews of their needs?
- How many people are missing out on accessing the AAC they need?
- How many people are self-funding their AAC?

Highlighting the impact of unmet need can be very powerful. Some examples of the impact of unmet need are as follows.

The impact on the person:

- Children without access to AAC are less able to access education and life opportunities.
- Adults without access to AAC are less able to engage in employment.
- People without access to AAC are more likely to experience social isolation and reduced quality of life.
- Not being able to have their communication aid maintained means people are going without a voice.
- People and their families experience an unclear pathway to achieving AAC, having to navigate multiple service and care pathways causes additional stress.
- People and their families have to apply for charitable funding, or self-fund, without an unbiased assessment from a practitioner.

The impact on practitioners:

- Practitioners spend significant time navigating routes to achieve funding (e.g., charity applications).
- Practitioners spend time dealing with complaints from service users.
- Practitioners feel unsupported without access to appropriate training or supervision.

(Adapted from "A proposed care pathway". AAC in South Yorkshire, Clarke et al. (2022) for The Barnsley Assistive Technology Team (unpublished).)

BOX 3.2 THE CHALLENGES OF MAINTAINING CARE PATHWAYS BY FIONNUALA O'DRISCOLL, SPEECH AND LANGUAGE THERAPIST

Care pathways are difficult to maintain when there are so many different services with different time frames for intervention involved.

Providing the stories of service users can be very impactful. Consider giving examples of stories where the appropriate AAC was provided and the impact this had, as well as examples of stories where the outcome was not so good and what this meant for the person.

The Ace Centre in the UK have provided some videos on their website which highlight the benefit of AAC: https://acecentre.org.uk/people-we-support

Outline what is required

What is needed to fill the current gaps in the service? Spend some time working out what resource you will need. This includes;

- Workforce: What practitioners do you need? How many and what will that cost?
- Equipment: What will this cost?
- Buildings and facilities: What space is required for the team and the equipment? Think about the space required to store equipment.

Approach the funding providers

Once you have gathered the data on prevalence, unmet need and impact, you can approach the person or people who have responsibility for funding services, often referred to as commissioners. Find out who the key people are and the best way to approach them. Some might be contactable directly, or perhaps there is a process in place for raising concerns. It might be easier to approach another service manager first, who might be better placed to have this conversation.

The Royal College of Speech and Language Therapists in the UK have produced a document "Resource Manual for Commissioning and Planning Services for SLCN" (Enderby et al., 2013) which gives some helpful guidance:

https://rcslt.org/wp-content/uploads/media/Project/RCSLT/slcn-resource-manual.pdf

Commissioners may expect to be presented with a proposed service specification, although this will likely be after the initial discussion. The document "Augmentative and Alternative Communication Services: Quality Standard for Commissioners" (Communication Matters, 2022) is helpful for providing a summary of why AAC services are required. Presenting a suggested care pathway, as included earlier in this chapter may also be helpful.

www.communicationmatters.org.uk/wp-content/uploads/2019/02/aac_quality_standard_for_commissioners_sept_2011.pdf

Summary

A good AAC service is one that meets the ongoing and changing needs of each person that needs to use it. Services must consider each stage of the care pathway and ensure that adequate funding is available, along with clear processes and procedures to support each stage of the pathway.

It is important to understand that AAC support is cyclical and never simply a case of providing equipment once. Ongoing management of equipment is vital.

The people supported by the service should know what they can expect from that service. Any interactions between services should be seamless, without gaps in support. Returning to a service (or services) should be easy.

Practitioners who are wanting to develop their service should first identify the need for the service by mapping their local population, considering those at risk of healthcare inequalities. Collecting data on who is likely to benefit from the service and highlighting the level of unmet need can be beneficial in helping those providing funding (commissioners) to see the impact on both service users and practitioners.

References

Clarke, Z., Judge, J., Robinson, H. (2022), AAC in South Yorkshire, The Barnsley Assistive Technology Team, unpublished.

Communication Matters, Augmentative and Alternative Communication (AAC) Services' Quality Standard for Commissioners (September 2011). www.communicationmatters.org.uk/wp-content/uploads/2019/02/aac_quality_standard_for_commissioners_sept_2011.pdf.

Communication Matters, Augmentative and Alternative Communication (AAC) Service Standards, Version 1.2 (August 2012). www.communicationmatters.org.uk/wpcontent/uploads/2019/02/aac_services_standard_aug_2012.pdf.

Enderby, P., Pickstone, C., John, A., Fryer, K., Cantrell, A. and Papaioannou, D. (2013). Resource Manual for Commissioning Planning Services for Speech, Language and Communication Needs, RCSLT. https://rcslt.org/wp-content/uploads/media/Project/RCSLT/slcn-resource-manual.pdf.

Local AAC Services Commissioning Toolkit (2023, 14 March). https://localaactools.co.uk/.

McNaughton, D., Giambalvo, F., Kohler, K., Nazareth, G., Caron, J. and Fager, S. (2018). Augmentative and Alternative Communication (AAC) will give you a voice: Key practices in AAC assessment and intervention as described by persons with amyotrophic lateral sclerosis. *Seminars in Speech and Language*, 39(05), 399–415. DOI: 10.1055/s-0038-1669992.

NHS England (2023, 31 March). What are healthcare inequalities? www.england.nhs.uk/about/equality/equality-hub/national-healthcare-inequalities-improvement-programme/what-are-healthcare-inequalities/.

NHS Education for Scotland (2014) IPAACKS Informing and Profiling Augmentative and Alternative Communication (AAC) Knowledge and Skills. www.aacscotland.org.uk/files/cm/files/ipaacks.pdf.

Pert, S. (2023) *Working with Children Experiencing Speech and Language Disorders in a Bilingual Context: A Home Language Approach*. Routledge.

RCSLT (2024) Augmentative and alternative communication (AAC) – Guidance. Royal College of Speech and Language Therapists. Augmentative and alternative communication (AAC) – guidance | RCSLT.

The Barnsley Assistive Technology Team (2021). Assistive Technology Specialist Role – Competencies Framework. www.barnsleyhospital.nhs.uk/assistive-technology/files/2018/02/Assistive-Technology-Specialist-Role-Competencies.pdf.

Zisk, A. H. and Konyn, L. (2022, 13 October). How to talk about AAC and AAC users (according to them). The AssistiveWare Blog. www.assistiveware.com/blog/how-to-talk-about-aac.

PART II
The Positive AAC Framework

Helen Robinson

The Positive AAC Framework (Robinson, 2023) was created to encourage a holistic view of AAC, recognising the interplay between many elements which, if supported well, can result in a positive experience of AAC.

There are six strands in the framework: Practice and Play, Preferences, Provision, Planning, People and Pride. There is no hierarchy or order to the strands.

Each strand has four dimensions and each dimension has a statement for consideration. Each strand is accompanied by two core values.

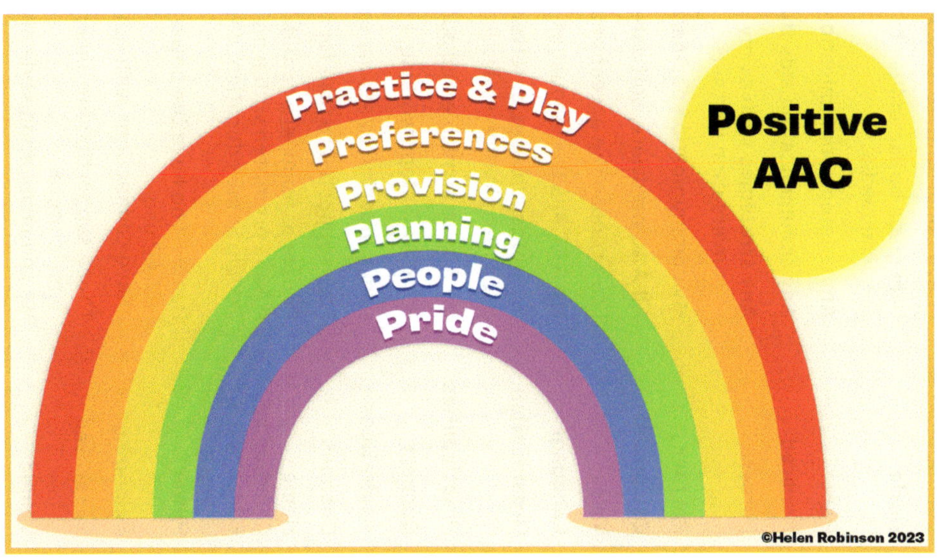

The Positive AAC Framework
Robinson, 2023.

DOI: 10.4324/9781003412311-5

Table 3.1 The Positive AAC Framework strands

Strand	Element	Statement	Outcome
Practice & Play	**Access**	I have opportunities to practice the ways I will access my AAC (e.g., eye pointing, scanning, switches).	**Real World**
	Control	I am given choice over the words & phrases added to my AAC and am show how to find them.	
	Communication	I have opportunities to explore how to use the words, phrases, or letters within my AAC system.	**Really fun**
	World	I am given opportunities to use my communication aid for things other than talking, e.g., TV control or social media.	
Preferences	**Paper**	Any printed communication resources are valued by my conversation partners.	**All equal**
	Powered	Any communication aids that have a voice output are valued by my conversation partners.	
	Person	Any strategies such as my voice, body, facial expression, gestures or signs are valued by my conversation partners.	**All valuable**
	Partner	My communication partners know how to support me to have a good conversation.	
Provision	**Equipment**	All AAC hardware, software, access methods and mounting are available to me.	**Always available**
	Voice	I can choose the accent and gender I want and/or have access to banked and synthetic voices.	**Always personalised**
	Language	My AAC has the languages that are used within my home.	
	Organisation	My words, phrases or letters are organised on my AAC system in a way that works for my communication style.	
Planning	**Practicalities**	My AAC is available and adapted as needed across different environments.	**My choice**
	Support	If my AAC stops working, I can get the help I need to fix it.	**My voice**
	Aspirations	I am supported to set my own goals and outcome measures for using my AAC.	
	Changes	I am supported to plan for transitions in my life and how my AAC may need to change.	
People	**Home**	People at home are confident in supporting me to use my AAC.	**Promoting awareness**
	Community	AAC is promoted within my local community and beyond. I can communicate wherever I go.	**Promoting acceptance**
	Education & Work	People in my education, day care setting or workplace are confident in how to support my AAC use.	
	Power	People who have the power to influence my AAC options have the right knowledge & skills to guide my AAC use.	
Pride	**Belonging**	I have connections with other people, who may or may not be disabled or use AAC.	**Everyone equal**
	Respected	Those supporting me understand & respect differences in how disability and AAC are viewed within my culture.	**Everyone heard**
	Valued	My communication style might be different and this is understood and accepted by others.	
	Promoted	People in positions of influence are aware of AAC and the barriers I might face in society.	

Source: Robinson, 2023.

AAC users and those who support them were consulted during the development of this framework. The rainbow and sunshine graphics were selected after consultation with practitioners and AAC users, asking them to suggest imagery that evoked feelings of positivity for them. Although these graphics might lend themselves towards a younger age group, the framework is intended to be applicable for all ages.

Part II of this book uses the framework to guide people working with AAC through the strands with the aim of providing a comprehensive guide to supporting AAC users and contributing towards a positive experience of using AAC. Photocopiable posters for each strand are available in the appendices.

Reference

Robinson, H. (2023). The Positive AAC Framework, Poster Presentation, Communication Matters Conference 12 September, 2023.

4

PREFERENCES

Helen Robinson

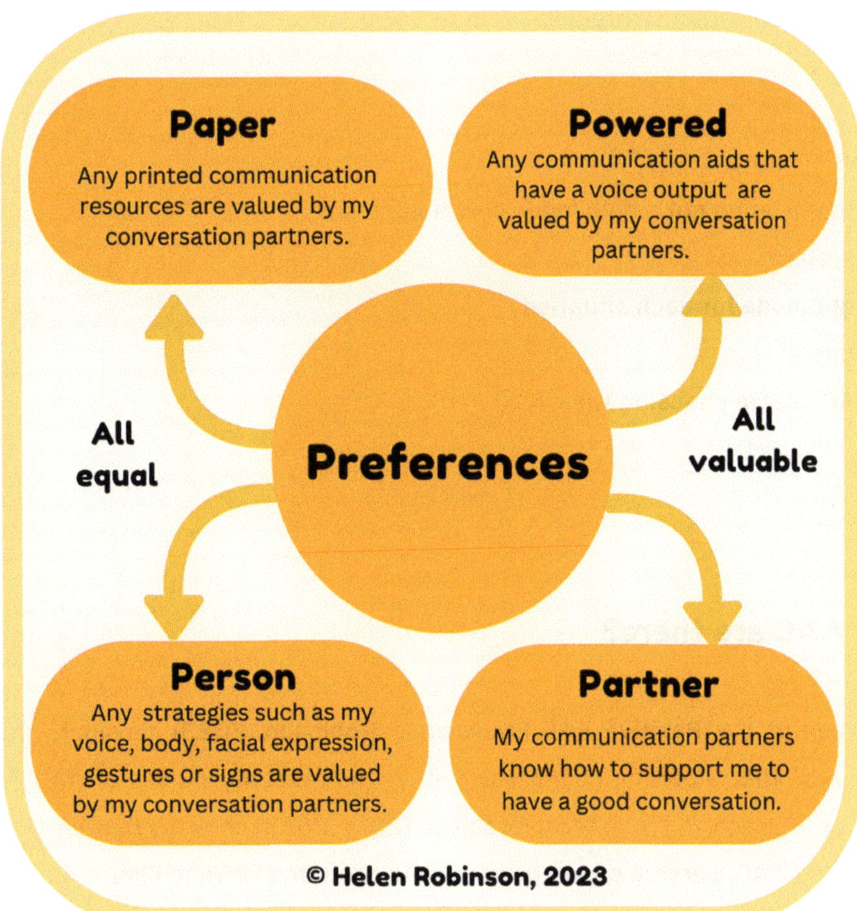

Figure 4.1 The AAC Preferences strand from The Positive AAC Framework
Source: Robinson (2023).

DOI: 10.4324/9781003412311-6

What types of AAC are there?

The preference strand of The Positive AAC Framework (Robinson, 2023) considers the types or modes of AAC that a person might use. Rather than classify modes of AAC as aided and unaided, or low tech and high tech, Robinson (2018, 2023) chooses to offer four categories for grouping AAC; person, paper, powered and partner, shown in Figure 4.1.

Person-based communication strategies

Person-based communication strategies are the ways a person can communicate using their body. This includes:

Speech and vocalisations

When considering AAC users, speech may often be forgotten as a potential mode of communication, however many AAC users will use speech in some situations. Some people refer to themselves as a "part-time" AAC user, or as "semi-speaking" for example, autistic people who may use speech sometimes, but at other times be unable to.

Clarke et al. (2023) found that people with dysarthria will show a preference for using speech above all other modes of communication, even if their speech is deemed unintelligible.

Vocalisations might be involuntary or voluntary sounds. Involuntary sounds include sneezing, coughing, hiccupping and snoring. Voluntary vocalisations are sounds such as laughing, crying, moaning and yelling. Some people may use approximations of spoken words, which are only understood by familiar communication partners (Beukelman and Mirenda, 2005).

Eye pointing

Sargent et al. (2013) describe eye pointing as:

> The context-relevant, controlled and intentional use of sustained gaze in order to direct one or more partner's visual attention to any item or object for a deliberate communicative purpose. Other communication modes (facial expression, vocalisation, head movement and body position) may be employed, as available, to support the use of gaze. The intended meaning is established collaboratively between the child and the adult.
>
> *(p. 479)*

Eye pointing might be used not just by children but by people of all ages with a range of diagnoses. Eye pointing can be particularly successful for people with severe physical impairments and medical conditions which cause them to fatigue easily and are therefore less likely to use powered communication aids which can be effortful (Beukelman and Mirenda, 2005).

Manual gestures and signing

Gestures are movements of that body such as facial expressions, hand movements and postures. They might be used for a range of functions;

- To convey a message, e.g. nodding for "yes".
- To emphasise spoken words, e.g. pointing to something while saying "look!"
- To display emotions (such as raising a hand to the mouth when shocked).
- To regulate a conversation for example nodding and maintaining eye contact to encourage the speaker to continue.
- To help with self-regulation (e.g., drumming fingers on a desk, playing with one's hair or chewing on a pen (Beukelman and Mirenda, 2005)).

Sparaci, et al. (2021) define three categories of gestures:

Deictic gestures: those which are used to draw attention to something in the environments often with the function of showing, giving or requesting; for example, pointing.

Representational gestures: those which indicate objects or actions not present or currently happening. For example, raising hand to mouth to indicate drinking or a drink.

Conventional gestures (a sub-group of representational gestures): those which convey specific linguistic meaning. For example, waving to convey "good bye" or "hello". These are often culturally specific.

Gestures are commonly used as part of multimodal communication by people without communication difficulties or differences. For people with cannot rely on speech to communicate all of the time, gestures or manual signs may provide an effective way to augment their speech, or as an alternative to spoken language.

For some AAC users, their gestures might be idiosyncratic and only understood by familiar communication partners. Physical impairment or apraxia may result in approximations of gestures or versions specific to the individual. Autistic children may develop gestures differently to non-autistic children, although studies have shown conflicting outcomes. Differences in gestural development may be influenced by apraxia which can be experienced by autistic people, and/or visuo-perception skills or sensory processing differences (Sparaci, et al., 2021).

People with Down syndrome will use manual signs as both alternative and augmentative communication. They will often use a sign to augment their spoken language, combining a sign and a spoken word to form a two-word message. There use of signs might be relatively short for some children acquiring spoken language, and for others they will go on to use signing as a means of augmenting their communication throughout their life (Launonen, 2021).

There is a distinction between gestures and signs (or sign language). Loncke (2021) describes sign language as "fully fledged linguistically organised systems" which "contain a lexicon, have formational (phonological) and combinatorial (morphological and syntactic) rules" (p. 24). Continuum theories propose that, at one extreme, gestures convey no lexical meaning whatsoever (such as hand movements accompanying speech), and at the opposing extreme they have clear linguistic use (for example, "thumbs up" for "yes").

Often, tradition and practitioner knowledge are reasons why children are taught gestures or signs as an alternative form of communication. Detailed assessment of the child's motor and linguistic skills is essential before choosing to introduce signing, as it may not be the most successful mode of communication. Practitioners must consider what is driving them to introduce signing over other modes of AAC (von Tetzchner, 2021).

Paper-based communication strategies

Paper-based aided communication has many advantages. It is relatively low cost and quick to produce and easy to amend or add to. Often favoured for being able to be used across many environments where powered communication aids might not be able to be taken, as shown by the example in Figure 4.2. and described in Box 4.1. Despite the flexibility of paper-based AAC, it can often be abandoned once powered communication is introduced, as described by speech and language therapist Emily Singleton in Box 4.2.

BOX 4.1 A QUOTE FROM FIONNUALA O'DRISCOLL

I think families still feel that a digital device can 'unlock' communication skills in a way that paper can't. Personally, I find using paper AAC much easier and more adaptable to different situations, e.g., using a PODD© book in a swimming pool or floor programme.

Fionnuala O'Driscoll, speech and language therapist

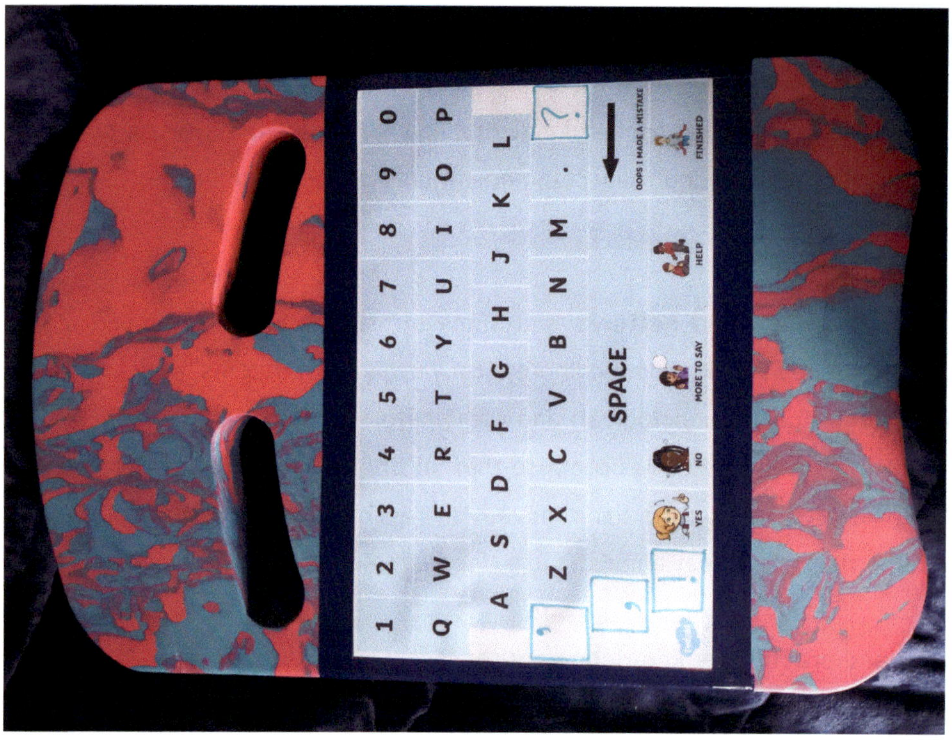

Figure 4.2 A communication board on a swimming pool float.
Source: Palframan and Jannikos (2023). Credit given to Emma Maskell-Ludlow for the idea.

Single page AAC displays

Single sheets of paper or card, often laminated for durability, are frequently used by people who require AAC. These pages might display photographs, graphic symbols, the alphabet or whole words or phrases. Often referred to a communication boards, these pages are often activity based when using photos or graphic symbols, for example snack time in school. For those who can use the alphabet, they can provide a low-cost, quick to produce communication method.

Communication books

Paper books with photographs, graphic symbols or text and common modes of aided communication. The way in which the photos, graphic symbols or text are organised within these books varies and is detailed in Chapter 5.

PECS

The Picture Exchange Communication System (PECS) was developed by Andy Bondy and Lori Frost in 1985. It has frequently been used with autistic children PECS uses six stages to teach children to exchange a graphic symbol or photograph for a desired item or activity. People might have a PECS book which pages with Velcro to attach cards with single graphic symbols or photographs. PECS is an intervention approach and not strictly a mode of AAC, however it is included in this chapter because it is often referred to amongst practitioners as a type of aided communication.

Although still widely used, there is a growing number of practitioners moving away from this approach in response to requests from members of the autistic community. Concerns have been raised about the use of physical prompting, where the adult places their hand over the child's and guides them to pick up the symbol and hand it to another adult in exchange for an item. Hand over hand prompting violates the child's body autonomy and causes frustration when the desired item is withheld. The PECS approach focuses on requesting or commenting, which is restrictive and does not allow the child to develop language in a flexible way (Lees, 2023).

E-Tran

Eye transfer, or E-Tran frames, are often made of transparent Perspex, with a cut-out in the middle for the user and their communication partner to see each other. Graphic symbols, photos, words or letters are placed in the corners of the frame on each side. The communication partner observes the eye pointing of the user to receive their message.

Eye link frames

Similar to E-Tran frames, eye link frames use sheets of Perspex but without the central cutout. Printed graphic symbols, words or letters can be stuck onto the frame, or these might be etched on if facilities are available. The communication partner holds the frame while the AAC user focuses on their chosen item. The partner then moves the frame around until their eyes meet the gaze of the AAC user. The selected message is then confirmed by the communication partner.

BOX 4.2 THOUGHTS ON PAPER-BASED AAC

I feel that people place a higher value on power-based AAC, though when this is given, they can find it the most overwhelming. I find that parents place less value on non-speaking systems (use of facial expression, gesture, pointing) and are often desperate for their young person to be moving onto what they feel is the next step. Paper- based systems often are most easy to implement but often when students change class, seem to be the ones that are disregarded the quickest.

Emily Singleton, speech and language therapist

Powered communication aids

Powered communication aids are often separated into those which use recorded speech and are battery powered (also known as lite or mid tech) and those which use synthesised speech and are mains powered (high tech). Collectively, they might also be known as voice output communication aids (VOCAs) or Speech Generating Devices (SGDs), which is then often shortened to "device".

Single message communication aids

These will aften use recorded speech, and are so-called because they can record a single message. **Big Mack switches** (see Figure 4.3) are commonly used, although many other types are available. Often thought of as an introductory form of AAC, they are actually useful devices for many AAC users. For some people who do not always have their paper or powered communication aids available in front of them, activating a single message device with a message that requests their AAC can be really helpful.

Single message communication aids are relatively low cost. There are a range of products to choose from, which will vary in terms of recording time, how to attach the labels and the type of battery/batteries required. Some of these devices will have additional features such as the ability to connect to switch adapted toys and appliances to control them.

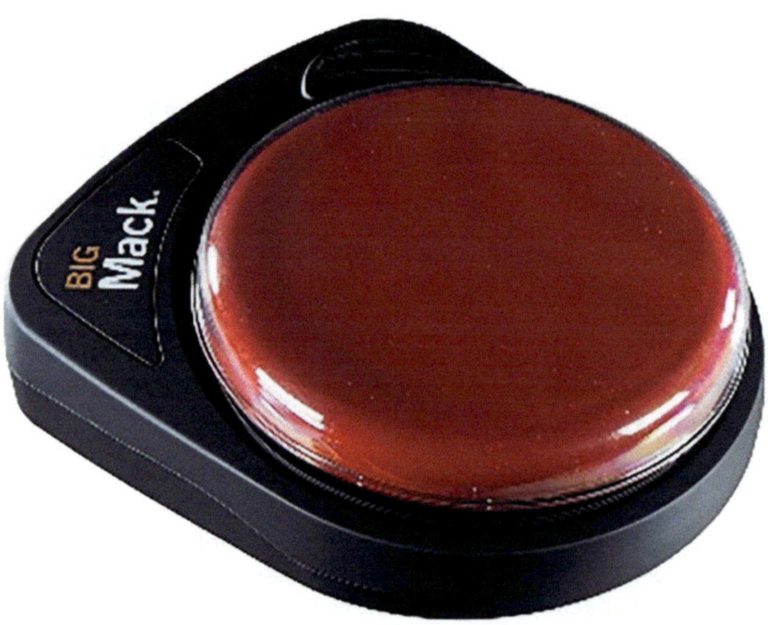

Figure 4.3 A Big Mack switch
Source: www.ablenetinc.com.

Message sequencer communication aids

Message sequencers are often one switch (button) that can store multiple messages. Many will have the option to plug an alternative switch into them if the user isn't able to press the message sequencer directly. These devices will have various modes to choose from. They will all offer the ability to move through a sequence of recorded messages. Some might have the function to play these messages back in a random order. This function might be used if the communication aid was being used to attract attention. Rather than saying "come here" every time, the messages can vary between "hi there!" "Come talk to me" and "I've got something to say".

Some message sequencers offer other functions, such as auditory prompts, where a second switch is plugged in and pressed to listen to the messages in a quieter voice. The user can use this to scan through the choices and when they find the message they want, they use the other switch to select and speak the message at a louder volume.

Static overlay communication aids

These communication aids will have a paper or laminated overlay (page) that has graphic symbols or text which is inserted into the communication aid (see Figure 4.4 for an example). Some **static overlay communication aids** might have a fixed number of messages, or there might be the option to change the number of messages by means of swapping the frame which sits on top of the overlay, for example moving from a grid of four messages to a grid of 12. These devices might have overlays with as few as two messages or over one hundred (see Figure 4.5 for an example).

The communication partner records their voice into each of the grid sections, also known as **cells**. Some static overlay devices will have multiple levels, to allow the communication partner or AAC user to switch the overlay for a different set of messages. For example, one overlay might have messages relating to a cooking class and the speech for this is recorded onto level 1. Another overlay might have messages about the library and the speech for this is recorded into level 2. Usually, a switch or a dial is used to change between the levels of recorded messages.

The AAC user selects the messages using direct touch or a switch. Some static overlay devices allow one switch to be plugged in for each message, so when each switch is pressed it speaks the corresponding message (up to eight switches and messages). Some devices have a "step-ahead" jack, which allows a switch to be plugged in and then as the user presses the switch the communication aid plays each message in turn.

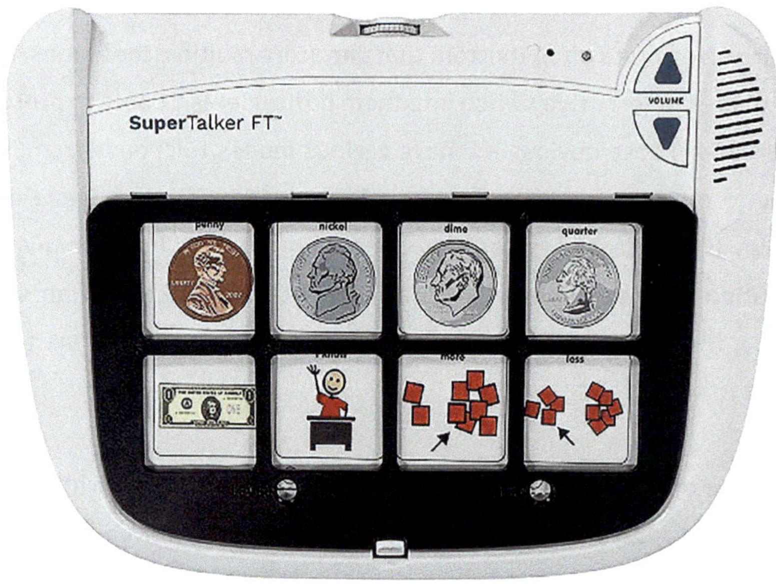

Figure 4.4 A SuperTalker communication aid

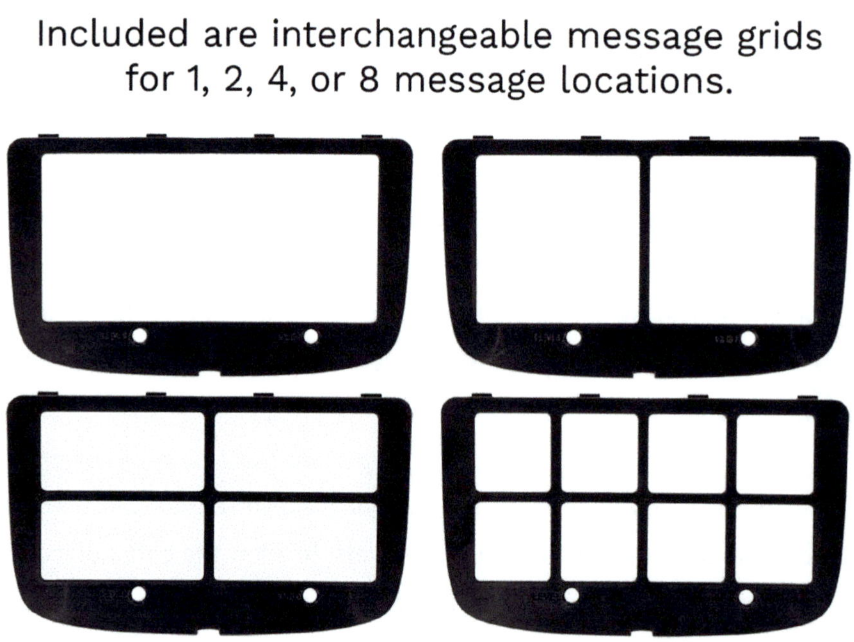

Figure 4.5 Four overlays for a SuperTalker communication aid

Tablet and computer communication aids

These are computers that use software to display graphic symbols, photograph or **alphabetical vocabulary packages.** The software might be an app on a tablet computer (e.g., an iPad), or it might be on a **dedicated device**, which is a communication aid produced and sold for the purpose of AAC. They are often referred to as **dynamic displays** because the messages change as the user selects them, for example selecting the cell labelled "people" will open a page of words relating to people. These are relatively high cost compared to other types of AAC.

These apps and software are often designed to offer vocabulary packages with tens or hundreds of pages which the user navigates through by selecting items which in turn lead to another page. However, as these apps and software are usually fully editable and customisable, they could also be used for relatively few messages, similar to a static overlay communication aid.

Tablet computer communication aids might be accessed, or controlled, by a range of methods which are outlined in Chapter 5. These devices are often viewed as being the preferred mode of AAC, and many people strive to acquire one. While they do offer much more in terms of available language and additional functionality such as environmental control and internet access (see chapter six), there are many reasons why a person might not prefer to use tablet or computer devices.

Clarke et al. (2023) reported that even people with unintelligible speech who are expert communication aid users will mostly use their communication aids "with strangers or in an unfamiliar environment and for communicative tasks to which the individual has ascribed a high level of importance" (p. 11). Other reasons might include effortful access methods (being difficult to use), limited battery life and restricted use in certain activities and environments such as the bathroom, outdoors, physical and messy activities.

Partner-based communication strategies

The relationship between the AAC user and their communication partner, in terms of how well they know each other, how confident and comfortable they feel and how equal they both feel, are important factors in the success of their interactions (Beukelman and Mirenda, 2002, 2015, cited in Midtlin et al., 2014). There is a body of evidence to show the benefits of communication partner skills training, especially for people with progressive and acquired communication difficulties. Broadly, the use of multimodal communication is shown to be beneficial (Volkmer et al., 2018). The communication partner can use a range of strategies to support the person with communication differences. These might include:

- Spoken and written key words
- Gesture and body language
- Hand drawings
- Photographs or graphic symbols

(Aphasia Institute, 2023)

Multimodal communication may also benefit people with developmental communication differences, along with multi-sensory referencing. This includes **sensory referencing, sensory queueing, tangible symbols** and **objects of reference**. These strategies are of particular benefit to people with learning disabilities or visual impairment (Talksense, 2023). The strategies discussed here are primarily for the purpose of supporting the individual's understanding of interactions. The skills of communication partners can also be used to support a person's expressive language. These include skills such as:

- Initiating and maintaining communication
- Turn taking
- Changing topics
- Repairing communication breakdowns

(von Tetzcher and Martisen, 2002; Beukelman and Mirenda, 2005, 2013 cited in Midtlin et al., 2014)

This chapter focuses on the multimodal communication strategies that communication partners can use to support a person's receptive language. The role of communication partners in supporting interactions will be further discussed in Chapter 6.

Referential objects

Referential objects, also known as objects of reference, can be used to support a person to understand what's happening. They are often used with people who are visually impaired. For example, a bangle might be used as a referential object for a teacher who always wears lots of jewellery. These objects can be used to give information about an activity that is about to happen. Often, objects will be multi-sensory, with a scent or texture that links to the activity or person. Miniature objects are sometimes used, for example a toy cow might be given to signify a trip to the farm. However, it can be challenging to make the link between these small items and the actual event. It is often a better idea to give an item with a clearer connection, such as using a piece of a swimming float to indicate that it's time to go swimming.

Tactile signing

Tactile signing, sometimes called **body signing**, is communication system that can be used to support a person's understanding, especially if they are visually impaired and have a limited understanding of spoken language. Tactile signing uses hand-under-hand signing or on-body signing. A popular approach used is Tactile Signing for Sensory Learners, known as **TaSSeLs** (Charnock, Woodall and Charnock, 2017).

Tangible symbols

Tangible or tactile symbols are 3 dimensional representations of words. These vary in how they are produced. It might be that a referential object is used, such as a Lego® piece being stuck onto a piece of card to represent the word "play" (Talksense, 2023). Other tangible symbols might be an exact copy of the graphic symbol, but use materials, like string or foam, to "raise up" the outline or shape of the symbol for the person to feel. Some tangible symbols might use shape and texture to identify the word category. The Project Core research team used 3D printed shapes in this way; verbs were triangles with vertical ridges, nouns were trapezoids with horizontal wavy grooves and adjectives were smooth heart shapes (Project Core, 2020).

Multimodal communication not single mode communication

The journey to becoming an AAC user, especially for people learning to use AAC from childhood, can often been seen as a linear one, introducing one mode and then another. At first, a person might be introduced to using objects or manual signing to support their communication, then progressing to use photographs and graphic symbols on a board or in a book. If they do well with these, they might be given a "mid tech" communication aid and if they succeed with this, they might eventually be given the opportunity to trial a "high tech" communication aid. A similar linear progression might also be applied to people with acquired communication difficulties, starting with an alphabet chart or graphic symbol book before trying a powered communication aid. There is a sense of "working towards" powered AAC, with the use of a voice output communication aid as the end goal. This linear, single mode model of progression between modes of AAC is shown in Figure 4.6.

There are understandable reasons why people would favour a linear progression through AAC modes, as shown in Figure 4.6. One obvious benefit is related to cost and available

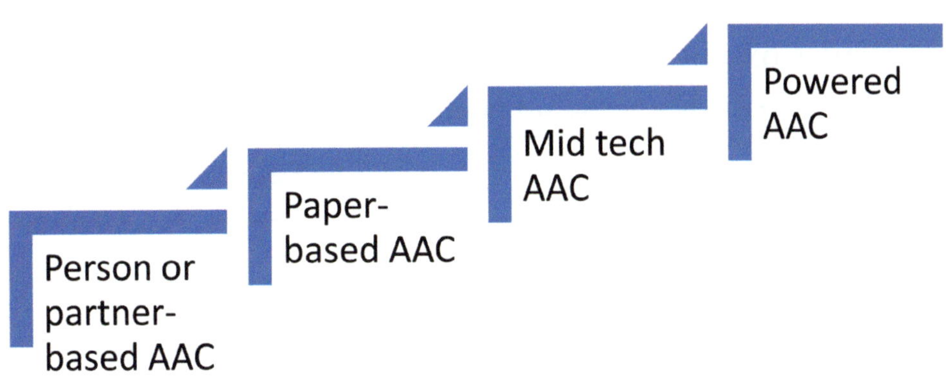

Figure 4.6 A linear, single mode model of progression through modes of AAC

resources. Powered communication aids are relatively expensive when compared to paper-based AAC. There is inevitably a tendency to require someone to demonstrate their skills with cheaper AAC methods prior to trialling higher cost powered communication aids and it's hard to imagine a world without some degree of linear progression through AAC modes.

The linear model of progression suggests the end goal as being the use of a powered communication aid, however neglecting other modes of AAC in the pursuit of powered communication may mean that the person misses out on the benefits of multimodal communication (Iacono et al., 2013 cited in Moran et al., 2023).

Studies have explored whether one mode of AAC is quicker to learn compared to others, for example manual signing compared to Picture Exchange systems, or Picture Exchange compared to powered communication aids (Beck et al., 2008; Bock, et al., 2005, cited in van der Meer, 2011.

A literature review by Sigafoos et al. (2003, cited in Sigafoos et al., 2005) concluded that there is no best AAC system and "recommended an individualized and evidence-based approach to identifying appropriate modes and systems when beginning AAC intervention" (Sigafoos et al., 2005, p. 143). A person's preference for AAC will depend on their individual characteristics and the environment they are in. This message is echoed in the I-ASC Exploratory model of clinical decision making (Lynch et al., 2019; Murray et al., 2019, companion papers).

The linear model of progression through AAC might mean that as they move from one mode to the next, the earlier modes are abandoned (Moran et al., 2023). There may be a tendency to see powered AAC as better and more desirable than other modes. For many AAC users, successful communication skills which they have spent months or years learning can be quickly neglected, as described by Carla Thompson in Box 4.3.

BOX 4.3 THOUGHTS ON MULTIMODAL AAC

> People think AAC is just high-tech devices and forget about all the other forms. They don't place as much value on them.
>
> *Carla Thompson, teaching assistant*

AAC does not need to begin with a particular mode. For some people, beginning with person, partner or paper-based AAC will not be appropriate. For people with visual impairments, paper-based AAC can be challenging (although many will find it helpful). For autistic people, powered AAC may be preferable (Lorah et al., 2022).

AAC does not need to include *all* the modes either. While multimodal communication is encouraged and used by many, some people may use relatively few modes.

Society promotes the idea that powered AAC is the best and other communication strategies are of lesser value. We should perhaps consider some of the drivers for this supposed ideal. Although without doubt the communication aid manufacturers and distributors are passionate about supporting people with communication difficulties and differences, they ultimately gain financially from the sale of powered communication aids. It's less easy to market and profit from paper, person and partner-based communication.

Families of AAC users who have struggled to use powered communication aids, or rejected them in favour of paper, partner or person-based AAC, may sometimes feel their loved one has "failed" in some way. Those who work with AAC users should consider their role in promoting all forms of AAC as having equal value.

A flexible AAC system

A person's preferences for one mode of AAC over another will change across contexts and communication partners and will reflect their changing needs across the day, week and year (Stafford et al., 2002, cited in van der Mer et al., 2011). Figure 4.1 shows the four modes of AAC: person, paper, partner and powered. A person might use some or all of these modes of AAC, and all have equal value and status.

Communication is likely to be multimodal, with the person utilising a range of AAC modes. Different modes of communication are likely to be combined across any given conversation, for example using a manual sign for one word and selecting a graphic symbol on a communication aid for another (Moran et al., 2023). Clarke et al. (2001) state that "children aim to maximise their communicative potential by combining modes of communication, and partners in interaction learn to recognise and respond to these strategies" (p. 108). Switching between modes of communication offers flexibility is likely to increase successful communication attempts. Each mode of communication will offer unique advantages in terms of accessibility, practicality and efficiency (Moran et al., 2023). In Box 4.4, AAC user Andrew describes his multimodal AAC.

BOX 4.4 ANDREW MAYERS DESCRIBES HIS MULTIMODAL AAC USE

I use the iPad where I can find the words from the pictures, able to pick from topics and categories. I also use the keyboard to write words, although it had to be changed to the alphabetic order as the qwerty was too difficult to find the letters. I use the white board option to draw. I use all of them, if I can't find the correct word, I can try finding the picture or I can try drawing it. One will definitely be working to get my message across.

Choosing the right mode for each situation

Clarke et al. (2023) explored the lived experiences of people with dysarthria and varying levels of speech intelligibility. Before considering how to communicate (the mode), they describe how a person must first decide whether to communicate at all. When considering if they should communicate, a person might ask themselves the following questions:

- Is the message important enough?
- How much time is available.
- Who is the communication partner?

If the person considers the effort of communicating to be worth it, they are then faced with the decision of *how* they communicate.

- How important is the message?
- How long will it take?
- Who is the communication partner?
- How do I prefer to communicate?
- How does my personality affect my communication?
- How am I feeling? (health or mood).

Clarke et al. (2023) discuss the important of prior experience on a person's choice of communication mode. Previous successful or unsuccessful communication attempts will influence each decision that is made, referred to as a communication loop. This loop is illustrated in Clarke et al.'s (2023) Model of communication with partially intelligible speech, shown in Figure 4.7. It helpfully illustrates that a person's preference for a particular mode of communication will change depending on a range of factors.

AAC users will likely prefer to have a range of AAC methods to choose from and assessment should allow the person to trial a number of options and indicate their preferred type of AAC. Sometimes it might not be clear why one type of AAC has been chosen over

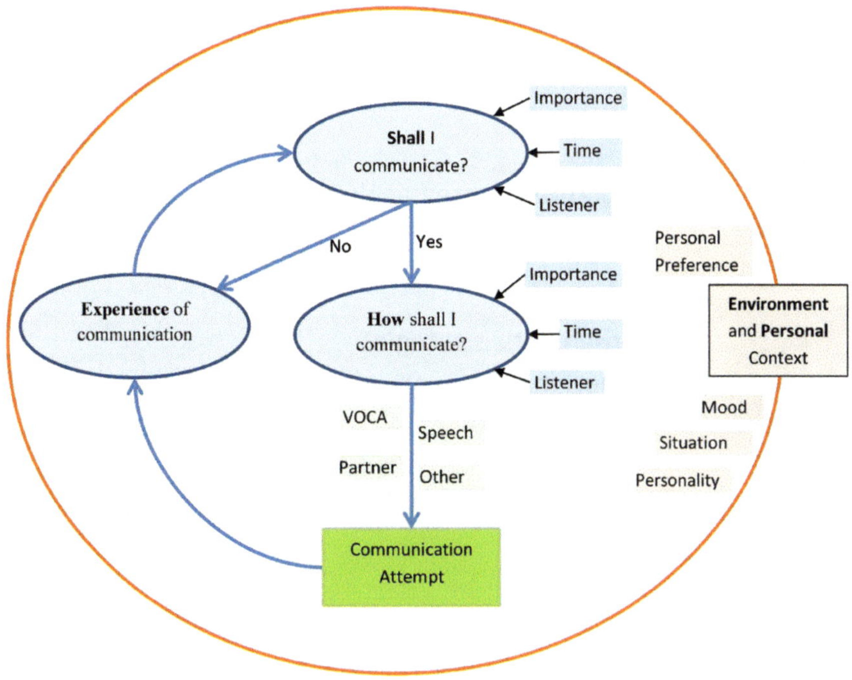

Figure 4.7 Model of communication with partially intelligible speech
Source: Clarke et al. (2023).

another. When comparing types of aided communication, preference might be related to factors such as the size, shape, voice or colour of the communication aid (van der Meer et al., 2011).

While the use of multimodal communication and its benefits is widely reported, there is little written about how people learn to use different modes of communication and how practitioners might support and encourage this. Moran et al. (2023) proposed a theory that the development of multimodal communication is inherent, taught and incidental, as shown in Figure 4.8. An observation checklist for a person's modes of communication is provided at the end of this chapter.

Part-time AAC users

There is growing acceptance that some people may only use AAC some of the time, which might be described as "part-time" AAC use. Their use of AAC might be related to the context, environment or communication partner(s). Some autistic people can use spoken words "some of the time, but not all of the time" (Zisk, 2022, 31 March) and refer to themselves as "semi-speaking".

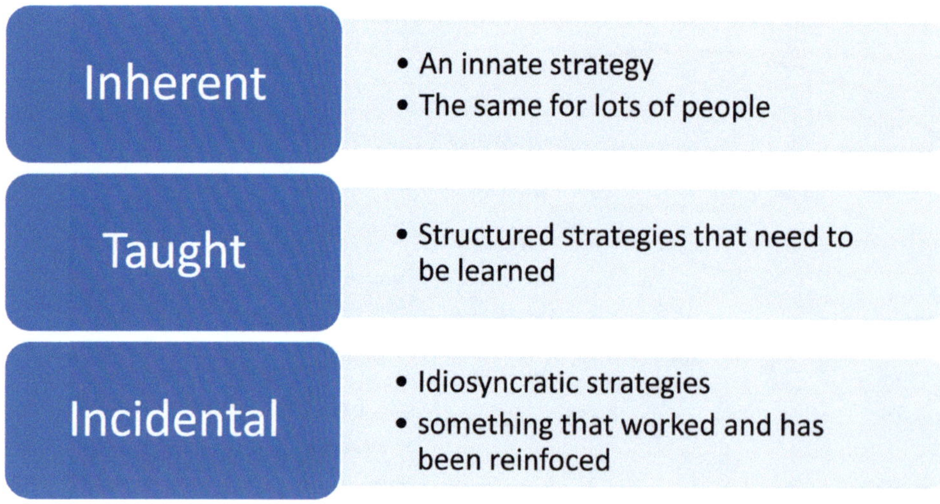

Figure 4.8 A theory about how multimodal communication strategies could be developed
Source: Moran et al. (2023).

Sometimes, the decision to use AAC in a situation might be planned ahead of time. This is more likely where the person knows they are going to be with communication partners who might not understand their communication and they will need to use alternative modes. Other times, the decision to use AAC might be more immediate, when speech suddenly isn't available. Here, Alyssa describes a scenario where they were able to predict that their speech might stop working and how they prepared to use AAC:

> Take yesterday for an example. Two of the lights in my building started to flicker, and completely predictably, this did a number on my ability to talk. A soon as I saw the first light, I reported it (seriously those are a safety risk, photosensitive epilepsy exists, my [*sic*] losing speech is nowhere near the worst thing that could happen because of a flickering florescent.) I also knew that I needed to make sure I had a workable communication method other than speech at all times for the rest of the day. As it turned out, speech stuck around until about 1pm, then I got it back briefly around 2:40. It went Kaput again right before 3 and came back around 4, after which it was iffy but extant for the rest of the day. Two of the three no-speech hours, I wrote on a white board to communicate. Writing on a white board is definitely my most used AAC.
>
> *Source: Zisk, 2015, 31 October.*

It is important to understand the fluctuation in a person's communication abilities and their ability and requirement to use different modes of communication. AAC users may vary between using the alphabet and graphic symbols. There is a tendency for practitioners to assume that because a person has the ability to use speech, that AAC is not required. Spoken language is prioritised as the superior mode of communication within society and among practitioners. All modes of AAC should hold equal status among each other (Robinson, 2018), but also alongside speech. Multimodal communication should be both accepted, promoted and normalised from an early age. Assumptions should not be made that just because someone is able to use speech, this will be their preference at all times (Donaldson et al., 2023).

Involving the AAC user in choosing their AAC

An individual may have the means to engage in a discussion about their AAC preferences. For example, people with degenerative conditions who still use speech will likely be able to discuss their choices with ease. Others may have existing modes of AAC that allow them to present an opinion. For those without existing AAC, asking questions for them to respond with "yes" or "no" will be helpful, providing they have a means to indicate this.

People with communication differences and particularly those with physical impairments may not be consulted on their views. Assumptions will often be made both about their abilities and their opinions, which can lead to distress and inability to assert one's identity (Toogood, 2022). Clarke et al. (2001) highlight the validity of children's views in relation to their health care provision and cite a range of policy and literature arguing for their consultation as part of good practice.

Seeking the opinions of people with learning disabilities can be challenging (Sigafoos et al., 2005). A literature review by van der Meer et al. (2001) reviewed seven studies involving AAC users with learning disabilities and identified an increase in the number of studies exploring AAC users' preferences over a 16-year period. The studies investigated by van der Meer et al. (2001) suggested that offering individuals two or more modes of communication and recording their selection across repeated occasions might be a reliable method of determining their preference. This approach is referred to as a "preference assessment approach" or "self-determination". This approach lends itself to choosing between two or more types of aided communication, such as three different powered communication aids, or between a powered communication aid and a paper communication book. It may be harder to use this approach when considering a person's preference for unaided communication strategies such as manual signing (Sigafoos et al., 2005). The available resources, such as time, finances and practitioner knowledge may limit the number of types of AAC that it is possible to trial and may be one reason why choices are made without offering the user choices.

Involving people in decisions about their lives is known to increase their health and well-being and reduce the likelihood of a person becoming distressed because their needs are unmet (Steiner, 2017). Sigafoos et al. (2005) highlight the positive impact of the self-determination approach on educational and therapeutic outcomes and caution against decision making by practitioners alone. Offering the person a choice of AAC options and observing their preferences will increase the likelihood of them using AAC successfully (van der Meer, et al., 2001). If asked, people will usually have an opinion regarding their AAC use (Midtlin et al., 2014).

Sigafoos et al. (2005) warn against sequence effects when offering people a choice of aided communication. It is important to ensure the individual isn't simply selecting the most recently used method in a series of trials. It is important that individuals have:

- Equal amount of experience with each type of aided communication.
- Equal amount of teaching relating to the use of each AAC type.
- Use of each type of AAC is altered across sessions to avoid the sequence effect.
- Opportunities for free choice are presented, without practitioner bias.

Sigafoos et al. (2005) also advocate for a fifth condition, where the individual's preferred item is made harder to obtain, as a means of further testing the reliability of their perceived preference. The strategy of withholding or sabotaging is no longer promoted as it is disrespectful to the person (Braun, 2021).

The methods of seeking a person's preference described so far have assumed that existing solutions will be presented to them for consideration. Beyond this, we might seek to involve AAC users in the design of AAC modes, referred to as **User Centered Design** (UCD). UCD seeks the views of AAC users, their families and AAC practitioners during the product design stage. Seeking the opinions of those with communication differences can be challenging and this may be why AAC users are not typically consulted. Lack of consultation may be a contributing factor to the high rate of abandonment of communication aids (Waller et al., 2005). If AAC users are consulted in the design of their aids, this is likely to increase their sense of ownership of the AAC and increase the likelihood of a positive attitude towards its use. Functionality, performance and aesthetics are all features which are likely to contribute to a communication aid being accepted by an individual (Clarke et al., 2001) and manufactures should not underestimate the importance of including the views of those who use them during the design stage.

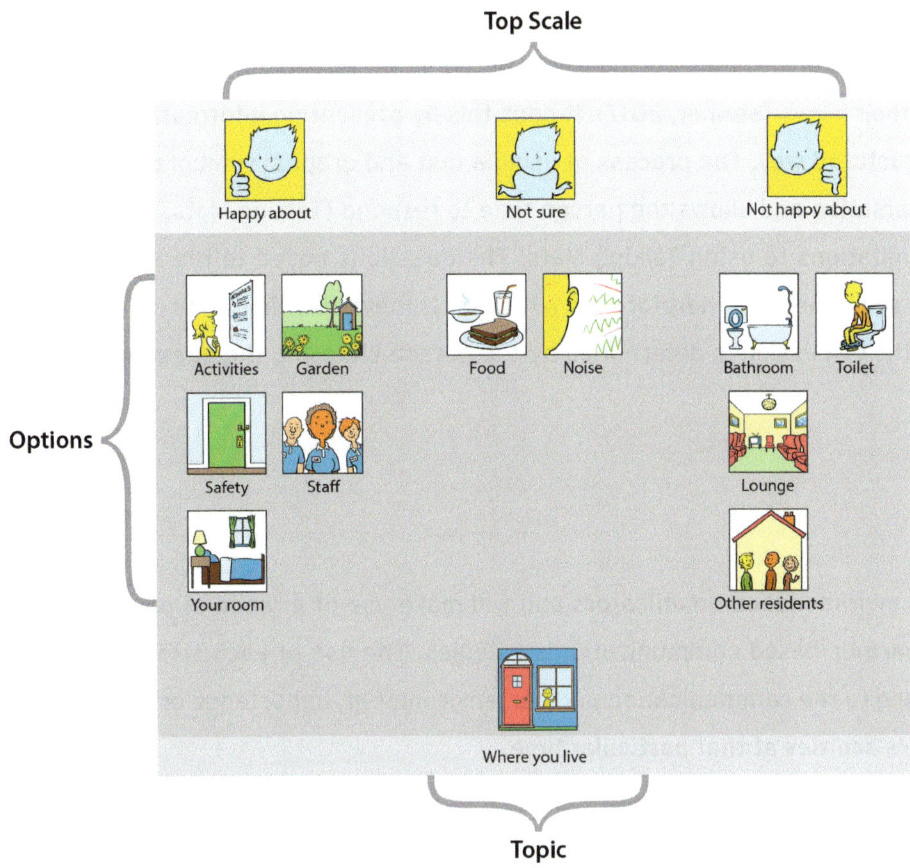

Figure 4.9 An example of a digital Talking Mat. The Symbols are designed and © to Adam Murphy 2015 and assigned to Talking Mats Ltd. in perpetuity. They may not be reproduced without permission. www.talkingmats.com

Talking Mats

A **Talking Mat** is a visual communication framework which helps practitioners to gain the views of people with communication differences (Stans et al., 2019; Broomfield, 2022). A Talking Mat can be a physical resource (a mat and graphic symbol cards) or an app on a tablet or computer. Each mat uses three sets of graphic symbols, for the topic, the options (choices) and a visual ratings scale (see Figure 4.9). A topic is chosen and the communication partner then gives the person the options in turn. The person either places the option along the rating scale, or indicates to the communication partner where to place it for them.

Resources for both the physical Talking Mats and the digital app can be purchased from www.talkingmats.com and there are training packages to demonstrate how to use them.

A number of studies have looked at the benefits of using Talking Mats (Hayden et al., 2023). Talking Mats have been shown to increase engagement, support the person's understanding of the issues being discussed (Midtlin et al., 2014) and increase their ability to express their views (Steiner, 2017). It does this by presenting information in smaller chunks in a structured way. The process of using a mat and graphic symbol options slows down the conversation and allows the person time to respond (Talking Mats, 2023). There are however limitations to using Talking Mats. The questions posed to the AAC user are determined by someone else, therefore the AAC user is inevitably limited to an extent and the quality of the discussion is determined by the person choosing the questions (Midtlin et al., 2014).

Summary

AAC users are multimodal communicators and will make use of a range of person, paper, powered and partner-based communication strategies. The use of each strategy is likely to vary according to the communication partner, environment, importance of the message and the person's abilities at that particular time.

There may be a tendency for people supporting AAC users to facilitate the abandonment of previously used modes in favour of a new one. AAC users should be encouraged to continue using previously acquired skills in order to maximise their communication success.

SUPPORT MATERIAL

Checklist for preferred modes of communication			
Name:		DOB:	Date completed:
	How might the person use these strategies?	What activities or contexts would they use these strategies?	Who would the person use these strategies with?
Person			
Paper			
Partner			
Powered			

Example checklist for preferred modes of communication			
Name: *Jack Smith*		DOB: *12/04/1962*	Date completed: *07/07/2024*
	How might the person use these strategies?	What activities or contexts would they use these strategies?	Who would the person use these strategies with?
Person	*Jack can vocalise, point with his eyes and turn his head to look towards things.*	*Vocalise to get attention or indicate pain or discomfort. Turn his head to indicate an object or person e.g., turns towards face cloth and looks at carer to ask for face wiping.*	*Anyone, but especially carers who are not confident in using his powered communication aid.*
Paper	*Alphabet chart with partner assisted scanning.*	*When tired or frustrated with powered communion aid. When in respite as Jack does not take his communication aid.*	*Lisa (wife), carers (not all are confident to use it), respite centre staff.*
Partner	*Objects to offer choices* *Listing options for Jack to indicate yes.*	*Anytime throughout the day, or especially when his communication aid is not available.*	*Wife, children, carers. Anyone really!*
Powered	*Tablet computer with eye tracker.*	*For more detailed discussions Emailing friends and family Facebook and Instagram.*	*Family members mostly, some carers (Tony, Sheila, Sam). Also when he is alone to use email and social media.*

References

Aphasia Institute. (2023) Communication tools: Communicative access & supported conversation for adults with aphasia (SCA™). www.aphasia.ca/communication-tools-communicative-access-sca/#:~:text=Supported%20Conversation%20for%20Adults%20With%20Aphasia%20(SCA%E2%84%A2)%20is%20a,Body%20language%20and%20gestures.

Beukelman, D. R. and Mirenda, P. (2005). *Augmentative & Alternative Communication: Supporting Children & Adults with Complex Communication Needs* (3rd ed.). Paul H Brookes Published Co.

Bock, S., Stoner, J., Beck, A., Hanley, L., Prochnow, J. (2005). Increasing Functional Communication in Non-Speaking Preschool Children: Comparison of PECS and VOCA. Education and Training in Developmental Disabilities. 40.

Braun, C. (2021, December 12). Case study in neurodiversity-affirming care: A toddler with childhood apraxia of speech. *Therapist Neurodiversity Collective blog.* Case Study in Neurodiversity-Affirming Care: A Toddler with Childhood Apraxia of Speech – Therapist Neurodiversity Collective (therapistndc.org).

Broomfield, K. (2022). The Unspoken Voices Project: Using creative methods in public involvement with people who use augmentative and alternative communication (AAC). In A. Volkmer and K. Broomfield (eds) *Seldom Heard Voices in Service User Involvement: The How and Why of Meaningful Collaboration* (pp. 111–129). J & R Press Ltd.

Charnock, D. and Woodall, J. (2017). *TaSSeLs Tactile Signing for Sensory Learners* (2nd ed.). Pavilion.

Clarke, M., McConachie, H., Price, K. and Wood, P. (2001). Notes and discussion: Views of young people using augmentative and alternative communication systems. *International Journal of Language and Communication Disorders*, 36(1), 107–115. https://doi.org/10.1080/13682820119446.

Clarke, Z. C., Judge, S., Fryer, K., Cunningham, S., Toogood, J. and Hawley, M. S. (2023). A qualitative study exploring the effect of communicating with partially intelligible speech. *Augmentative and Alternative Communication*, 32(2), 110-122. https://doi.org/10.1080/07434618.2023.2206910.

Donaldson, A. L., Corbin, E., Zisk, H. and Eddy, B. (2023). Promotion of communication access, choice, and agency for autistic students. *Language, Speech, and Hearing Services in Schools*, Tutorial, 54(1). https://doi.org/10.1044/2022_LSHSS-22-00031.

Hayden, N. K., Bradshaw, J., Hayward, S., Murphy, J., Boa, S., Eden, V., Mischo, S., Pampoulo, E., Macrae, A.-M., Reid, J., Darvell, C. Lauer, N. Mundt, I., Clark, L., Nagawa, M., Duner, A. and Talking Mats Research Network (2023). Summary of Talking Mats studies. Talking Mats www.talkingmats.com/wp-content/uploads/2023/05/Summary-of-Publications-Featuring-Talking-Mats.pdf.

Iacono, T., Lyon, K., Johnson, H., & West, D. (2013). Experiences of adults with complex communication needs receiving and using low tech AAC: an Australian context. *Disability and Rehabilitation: Assistive Technology*, 8(5), 392–401. https://doi.org/10.3109/17483107.2013.769122

Launonen, K. (2021). Sign acquisition in Down syndrome: Longitudinal perspectives. In N. Grove and K. Launonen (eds) *Manual Sign Acquisition in Children with Developmental Disabilities* (pp. 195–212). Nova Science publishers, Inc.

Lees, E. (2023, 7 July). So what's wrong with PECS? www.autisticslt.com/pecs-aba.

Loncke, F. (2021). Manual signing and psycholinguistics. In N. Grove and K. Launonen (eds) *Manual Sign Acquisition in Children with Developmental Disabilities* (pp. 195–212). Nova Science publishers, Inc.

Lorah, E. R., Holyfield, C., Miller, J., Griffen, B. and Lindbloom, C. (2022). A systematic review of research comparing mobile technology speech-generating devices to other AAC modes with individuals with autism spectrum disorder. *Journal of Developmental and Physical Disabilities*, 34(2), 187-210. https://doi.org/10.1007/s10882-021-09803-y.

Lynch, Y., Murray, J., Moulam, L., Meredith, S., Goldbart, J., Smith, M., Batorowicz, B., Randall, N. and Judge, S. (2019). Decision making in communication aid recommendations in the UK: Cultural and contextual influencers. *Augmentative and Alternative Communication*, 35(3), 180–192. https://doi.org/10.1080/07434618.2019.1599066.

Midtlin, H. S., Næss, K-A. B., Taxt, T. and Karlsen, A. K. (2014). What communication strategies do AAC users want their communication partners to use? A preliminary study, *Disability and Rehabilitation*, 37(14), 1260–1267. https://doi.org/10.3109/09638288.2014.961659.

Moran, C., Randall, N. and Judge, S. (2023). How do people who use augmentative and alternative communication use multimodal communication in real- life situations? A literature review. *The Journal of Communications Matters*, 37(1), 26–29.

Murray, J., Lynch, Y., Meredith, S., Moulam, L., Goldbart, J., Smith, M., Randall, N. and Judge, S., (2019). Professionals' decision making in recommending communication aids in the UK: Competing considerations. *Augmentative and Alternative Communication*, 35(3), 167–179. https://doi.org/10.1080/07434618.2019.1597384.

Palframan, L. and Jannikos, M. [@ChocToothpaste]. (2023, 11 June). My daughter now has the smartest letterboard [tweet]. Twitter. https://twitter.com/ChocToothpaste/status/1667946128606633984.

Project Core. (2020, January). Universal Core Vocabulary - 3D Symbol format. www.project-core.com/3d-symbols/.

Robinson, H. (2018, March). AAC technology: What's in a name? *RCSLT Bulletin*, 11, 791.

Robinson, H. (2023). The Positive AAC Framework [Poster presentation], Communication Matters Conference, 12 September, 2023.

Sargent, J., Clarke, M., Price, K., Griffiths, T. and Swettenham, J. (2013). Use of eye-pointing by children with cerebral palsy: What are we looking at? *International Journal of Language & Communication Disorders*, 48(5), 477–485.

Sigafoos, J., Drasgow, E., Schlosser, R.W., (2003), Strategies for beginning communicators, in: The Efficacy of Augmentative and Alternative Communication: Toward Evidence-Based Practice, Schlosser, R.W., ed., Academic Press, Boston, Academic Press, Boston, pp. 323-346.

Sigafoos, J., O'Reilly, M., Ganzb, J.B., Lancioni, J.G. and Schlosser, R. D. (2005). Supporting self-determination in AAC interventions by assessing preference for communication devices. *Technology and Disability*, 17(3), 143-153.

Sparaci, L., Romana, F. L. and Capirci, O. (2021). More than words: Gestures in typically developing children and in children with autism. In N. Grove and K. Launonen (eds) *Manual Sign Acquisition in Children with Developmental Disabilities* (pp. 195–212). Nova Science publishers, Inc.

Stans, S. E. A., Dalemans, R. J. P., de Witte, L. P. and Beurskens, A. J. H. M. (2019). Using Talking Mats to support conversations with communication vulnerable people: A scoping review. *Technology and Disability*, 30(4), 153–176. https://doi.org/10.3233/tad-180219.

Steiner, N. (2017). A service level evaluation of the impact and effectiveness of Talking Mats as a consultation tool. www.talkingmats.com/wpcontent/uploads/2013/09/Report-from-CLCH.pdf.

Talksense (2023). *Multi-sensory Referencing and Objects of Reference*. https://talksense.weebly.com/oor.html.

Toogood, J. (2022). Enabling and empowering people with seldom heard voices in service user participation: A user perspective. In A. Volkmer and K. Broomfield (eds) *Seldom Heard Voices in Service User Involvement: The How and Why of Meaningful Collaboration* (pp. 13–23). J&R Press Ltd.

Volkmer, A., Spector, A., Warren, J. D. and Beeke, S. (2018). The "Better Conversations with Primary Progressive Aphasia (BCPPA)" program for people with PPA (Primary Progressive Aphasia): Protocol for a randomised controlled pilot study. *Pilot Feasibility Study*, 158 (4). https://doi.org/10.1186/s40814-018-0349-6.

van der Meer, L., Sigafood, J., O'Reilly, M. F. and Lancioni, G. E. (2011). Assessing preferences for AAC options in communication interventions for individuals with developmental disabilities: A review of the literature. *Research in Developmental Disabilities*, 32, 1422–1431. https://doi.org/10.1016/j.ridd.2011.02.003.

Von Tetzchner, S. (2021). Manual signs and graphic symbols as complimentary forms of augmentative and alternative communication. In N. Grove and K. Launonen (eds) *Manual Sign Acquisition in Children with Developmental Disabilities* (pp. 195–212). Nova Science publishers, Inc.

Waller, A., Balandin, S. A., O'Mara, D. A. and Judson, A. D. (2005). Training AAC Users in User-centred Design, Proceedings of the Accessible Design in the Digital World 2005 Conference, British Computer Society, London, England (pp. 1–7).

Zisk, A. H. (2015, 31 October). #AAC Awareness Month: When speech output isn't best. Yes, that too blog. http://yesthattoo.blogspot.com/2015/10/aac-awareness-month-when-speech-output.html.

Zisk, A. H. (2022, 31 March). The Intersectional Infinity Summit. Yes, that too blog. http://yesthattoo.blogspot.com/2022/03/the-intersectional-infinity-summit.html.

5

PROVISION

Helen Robinson

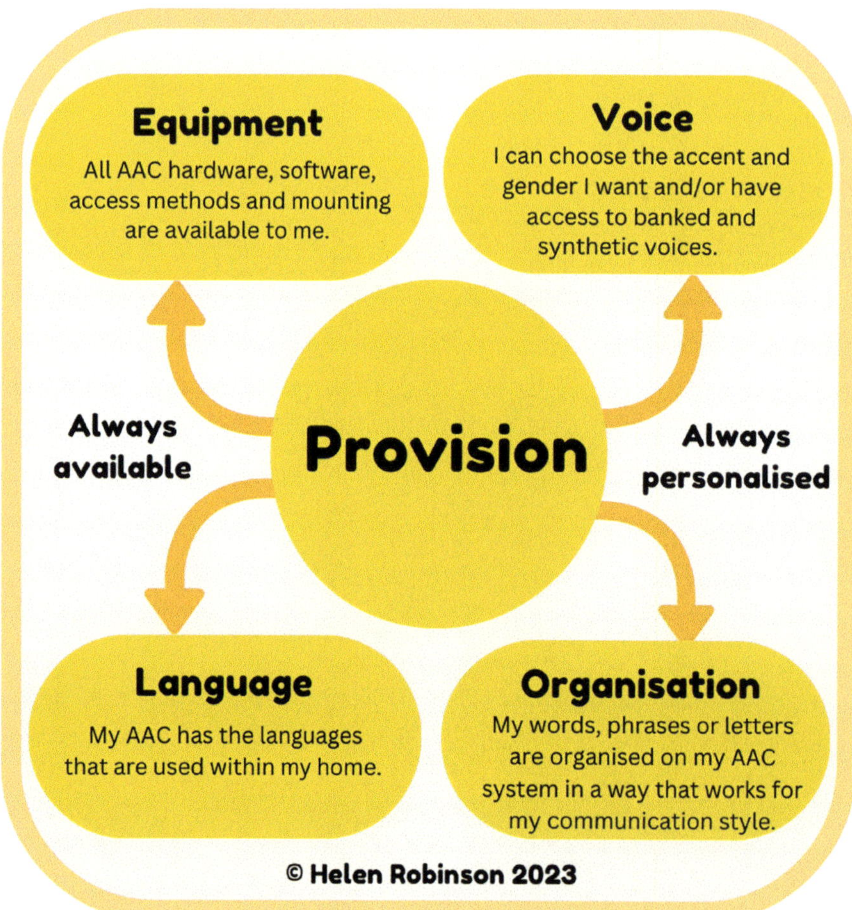
Equipment
All AAC hardware, software, access methods and mounting are available to me.
Voice
I can choose the accent and gender I want and/or have access to banked and synthetic voices.
Always available
Provision
Always personalised
Language
My AAC has the languages that are used within my home.
Organisation
My words, phrases or letters are organised on my AAC system in a way that works for my communication style.
© Helen Robinson 2023

Figure 5.1 The AAC Provision strand from The Positive AAC Framework
Source: Robinson (2023a).

- A robust AAC system

  Customisation

  Communication

  Another blog post by PrAACtical AAC suggests the following requirements:

DOI: 10.4324/9781003412311-7

This chapter considers the elements which need considering when providing someone with aided communication. The phrase AAC system is used widely and can refer to the features of one mode of AAC that a person uses (e.g., a paper communication book) or a collection of all their AAC strategies (e.g., eye pointing, an iPad with an app and an alphabet board).

Between 30%–50% of AAC systems are abandoned, often at great financial cost, yet the reasons for abandonment are not well understood. There is also "lack of robust evidence surrounding the decision-making process" (Webb et al., 2019, p. 2), but we do know that successful AAC use is more likely when the chosen AAC system meets the needs of the individual (Webb et al., 2019).

The four dimensions within The Positive AAC Framework (Robinson, 2023a) strand of "Provision" (see Figure 5.1) will serve as a guide to consider how we make choices about hardware, access methods, software, representational methods and organisational method/vocabulary.

A robust AAC system

The term "robust AAC" is now commonplace within the fields of AAC. This requirements of a robust AAC system were explored by Franco et al. in 2018. They proposed that developer of AAC systems should produce products which consider the two umbrella terms of "customisation" and "communication". Franco et al. (2018) detail both the requirements of robust AAC and the options to consider, summarised here as follows;

Customisation

1) **Vocabulary customisation.**
   a) The vocabulary selection: An extensive vocabulary using core and fringe words, alongside pragmatic functions of communication.
   b) The language representation method, which may be one of three options:
      i. Alphabet based: One concept is represented by a word.
      ii. Single meaning pictures: One concept is represented by one picture.
      iii. Semantic compaction: One concept is represented by a sequence of pictures.
   c) The vocabulary organisation, which may be one of two options:
      i. Taxonomic (categories e.g., food, people).
      ii. Contextual (schematic, e.g., by activity or place).
2) **Interface customisation**: The ability to change the visual, audio and other settings to make the AAC system accessible to the individual.

Communication

3) **Communication flexibility.**
   a) Freedom of communication to allow for Spontaneous Novel Utterance Generation (SNUG), by providing the user with single items which they can freely combine.
   b) Shortcuts to increase speed of communication: word prediction and pre-stored phrases.
4) **Appropriate audio and visual feedback, which might be done in two ways:**
   a) Per item selected whilst constructing a message.
   b) When the whole message is selected to be spoken aloud as one unit.
5) **Construction of meaningful sentences, which might be done in three different ways:**
   a) The theory of scripts (Todman et al., 2008, cited in Franco et al., 2018): Structured, predictable messages framed around an activity.

b) Prediction techniques: The AAC system predicts the user's next choice and offers a narrowing number of items to choose from.
c) COMPANSION system The AAC system takes the user's message and expands on it to offer a grammatically correct sentence (Demasco and McCoy, 1992, cited in Franco et al., 2018):

Further definitions of a robust AAC system can be found in abundance. A blog post by the AAC developer AssistiveWare defines a robust AAC system as including the following:

- Communication functions
- Core words
- Fringe and personal vocabulary
- Access to the alphabet
- Preprogrammed phrases and sentences.

(AssistiveWare, accessed 31 October 2023)

Another blog post by PrAACtical AAC suggests the following requirements:

- Multiple components (including voice, paper-based AAC, phones, white boards)
- Multimodal communication (including gestures and signs, objects, facial expression)
- Access to the alphabet
- Different types of words, which include; core and fringe vocabulary and preprogrammed phrases
- Flexibility in word forms (the ability to change the word endings)
- Thoughtful organisation
- Evolution: the ability for the system to expand.

(Zangari, 2021)

It is important to reflect on the range of definitions of a robust AAC system, given the extent to which this term is used by those working with AAC. While there is variation in the definitions, there is also commonality to be found.

In summary, a robust AAC system is one which provides a range of vocabulary, organised in a way which is meaningful to the user, has access to the alphabet and graphic symbols and is flexible and customisable.

Equipment

In this section, we shall consider the choices that need to be made around hardware, which refers to any AAC which isn't person or partner based. Chapter 4 has already looked at the types of AAC hardware that are available (e.g., tablets, dedicated devices, communication books, Etran frame, static overlays) and Chapter 2 explored the factors which need to be considered when choosing AAC (see Table 2.2 and "Assessment form for competing considerations"). Here, we shall look at ways of controlling a communication aid (access methods) and **mounting options**, if required.

Mounting

Mounting, or "a mount" refers to the equipment which holds a communication aid in place on either the floor, a wheelchair, table, armchair, bed or standing frame. Mounts for use on a table top or the floor (sometimes called a floor stand) are readily available. If the communication aid is going to be attached to a wheelchair, armchair, bed or standing frame, this may require a specialist practitioner to fit the mount due to the associated risks, some of which are outlined here;

- Risk of tipping: If the weight of the communication aid is not balanced, the mount can tip over.
- Risk of falling off: If the communication aid isn't securely fixed onto the mount, it can become unattached and fall on the floor or person.
- Risk of trapping: If mounted to a wheelchair, armchair or bed which can move, there is a risk of trapping the person's body parts between the communication aid, mount and wheelchair/armchair/bed.

Appropriate training for the people who will set up and operate the mount is important. Clear instructions should be easily available, which might be in picture, written or video format.

A mount is usually made up from the following components:

The base: This might be a frame clamp and tube socket if attaching to something. This is the part that the tube slots into and can usually be locked in place. If it's a table/desk or floor mount it might be a flat plate or a rolling base (on castors).

Tubes and joints: There is usually a vertical tube (sometimes referred to as a pole) and a horizontal tube, which holds the communication aid. Joints might be fixed, swivel, folding or 3D (allowing 360° movement).

The socket: This is the part the fits around the tube and holds the communication aid. There is often a quick release pin which is pulled to allow the communication aid to slide in and out. The socket can be fixed or might be adjustable via a handle, to allow the position of the communication aid to be changed.

The adaptor: This is often referred to as the "mounting plate" and is the part that fixes to the back of the communication aid. The adaptor slides into the socket and is held in place with the quick release pin.

If someone is using a **switch** to control/access their communication aid they might need their switch(es) to be mounted. Fixed or flexible mounts are available and can be clamped onto a wheelchair, table/desk, armchair or bed frame.

Mounts are also available for smaller items such as mobile phones. It's worth considering whether a person would benefit from their paper based AAC mounting too. This might require a more bespoke mounting solution as ready-made solutions are less readily available.

Mounts are not safe to use whilst in moving vehicles and other forms of AAC should be considered when travelling.

Access methods

AAC access methods allow a person to control their communication aid, or *access* it. They are often described as direct or indirect. Direct access methods are ones where the person uses a body part or a tool to point to something (such as an object, letter or graphic symbol). Indirect access methods are ones where the person uses scanning to move between choices before making a section. Descriptions of access methods are given in Table 5.1. For ideas to improve or practice access to AAC, see Chapter 6.

Types of switches

There are a wide range of switches available. The person needs to have a reliable, repeatable movement to be able to control a switch. Switches might be controlled by fingers,

Table 5.1 Descriptions of access methods

Access method	*Description*
Touch/pointing	The person uses a body part to make a selection e.g., finger, fist, nose, foot.
Keyguard/touch guide	Keyguards are plastic overlays that sit on the screen of a communication aid. Holes are positioned over each cell, for the user to put their finger through. Touch guides are similar but tend to be thinner. These can support people who might accidently press **cells** due to reduced hand function, or a tremor.
Stylus	Standard styli look like a pen and can support access to paper or a screen if pointing is tricky.
Light/laser pointer	Often worn on the person's head, attached via a headband or glasses, the light pointer is used to indicate a selection on paper-based AAC. Infrared light pointers can be used to control some power-based communication aids.
Head tracker	Head trackers are small devices which sit on the top of some power-based communication aids. The user wears a small reflective dot, usually on their forehead or glasses. Infra-red detects the person's head movements. Some software can track head movements without a peripheral head tracker. Apple iOS allows gestures, such as puffing cheeks or opening the mouth, to be assigned to a certain actions or messages.
Eye gaze/pointing	The person looks at their target and confirms their selection by dwelling on the item or blinking (powered communication aids), or looking back at their communication partner (paper communication aids). Power-based AAC uses infra-red eye trackers to track their eye movements. Some people who find dwelling or blinking tricky might use eye gaze to find their target and then use a switch to select it (combined access method).
Keyboard	People who can use the alphabet to spell might have difficulty using a touch screen, but manage a keyboard. Adapted keyboards are available, which might have bigger buttons or a keyguard over the top.
Joystick/trackpad/mouse	These can be used to control a curser on the screen. A selection can be made by pressing a button on the joystick, trackpad or mouse, or an additional switch might be used to make the selection.
Visual scanning	The communication partner points to items, or the powered communication aid scans through items. There are different scanning patterns (see Figures 5.5–5.8). The AAC user is familiar with the items on the screen so does not need to listen to an auditory cue. When their choice is reached, they indicate "yes" if it's a paper-based communication aid, or activate their switch if it's powered.
Auditory scanning	The powered communication aid reads aloud the options and the AAC user confirms their choice my activating their switch.
Auditory phishing	The user touches the screen and one voice reads aloud the items touched. A longer press on the screen will activate that item and a second voice speaks. Used by people with visual impairment.
Partner-assisted scanning	The communication partner reads aloud the options and the AAC user confirms their selection with their "yes" response.

hands, heads, knees, feet, toes, elbows, noses, sucking/blowing or blinking. Some switches can detect nearby movement but don't require contact to be made. This are known as proximity switches (see Figure 5.2). Switches can also be controlled using **electromyography (EMG)**, where a sensor is stuck to the person's skin and detects electrical impulses from muscle movements. EMG switches can be used where there is minimal muscle movement (Judge, Nasr and Hawley, 2018). Figures 5.2, 5.3 and 5.4 show examples of three commonly used switches.

Scanning patterns

The scanning pattern is the order in which the computer or person moves through the available choices, highlighting them as they are scanned. Highlighting might be a coloured frame around the item, speaking the item aloud, zooming in on the item or changing the colour of the cell.

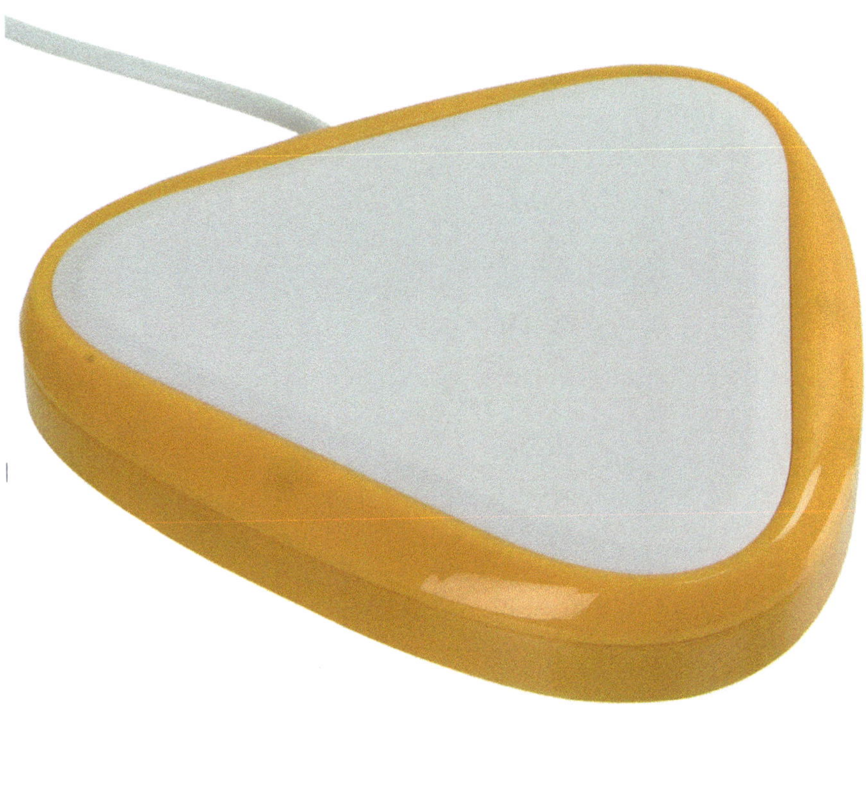

Figure 5.2 A candy corn switch from AbleNet, Inc.
Source: www.ablenetinc.com.

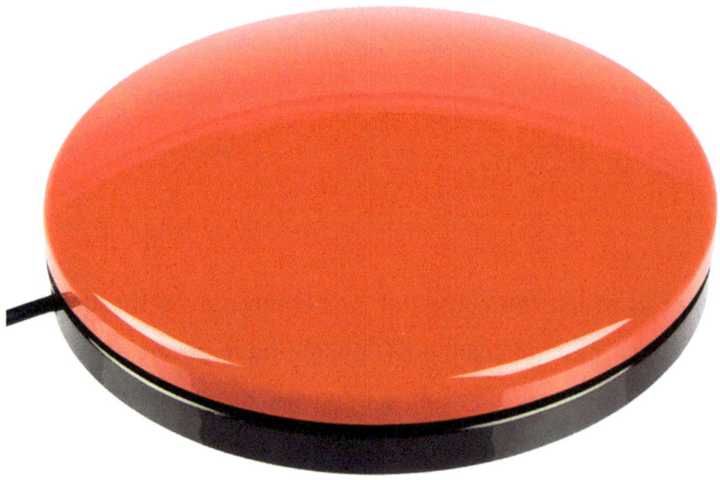

Figure 5.3 A buddy button switch from AbleNet, Inc.
Source: www.ablenetinc.com.

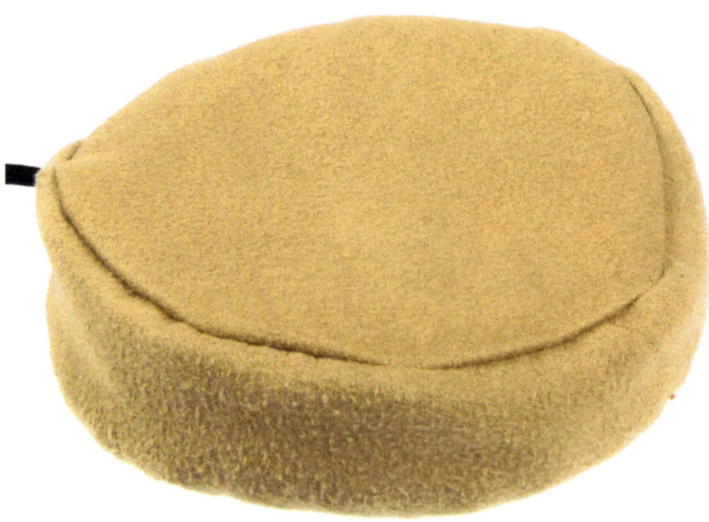

Figure 5.4 A pillow switch from AbleNet, Inc.
Source: www.ablenetinc.com.

The most common scanning patterns are described and shown here:

Single switch/item scanning: The person, or communication aid, moves through the items one at a time, highlighting them in turn. Sometimes called auto-scan (see Figure 5.5).

Two switch scanning: The person uses one switch to move between items and a second switch to select the one they want (one to move, one to choose). Sometimes called "step scanning".

Row-column scanning: The person, or communication aid, highlights one row at a time. When the user makes a selection, the scanning continues along the row (one column at a time). The user then makes a second selection to confirm their choice. This method requires the user to be familiar with the items on their communication aid but can be a useful method for increasing speed (see Figure 5.6).

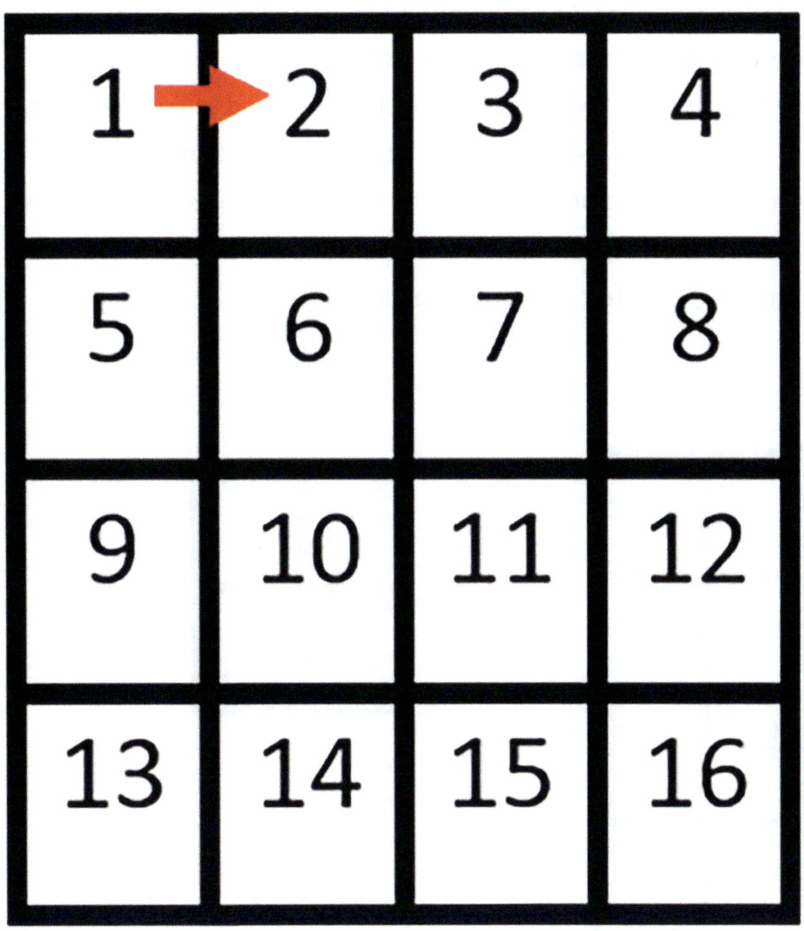

Figure 5.5 Diagram of single switch/item scanning

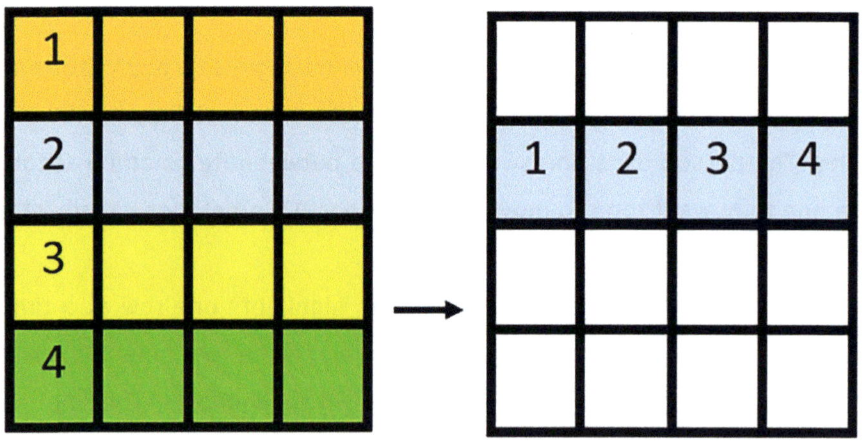

Figure 5.6 Diagram of row-column scanning

Block scanning: The items on the page are grouped into blocks. The communication partner, or the communication aid, highlights one block at a time. The user makes a selection and then the scanning continues, item by item, within the chosen block. The user makes a second selection to confirm their chosen item (see Figure 5.7).

Elimination scanning: This requires two switches, which correspond to two colours on the screen. Half the items on the screen are one colour and the other half another colour. Each time the user selects a colour (e.g., blue switch for the blue half of the screen) the choices are reduced by half. The items on the screen continue to be split into two colours and the user keeps pressing until only one item remains (see Figure 5.8).

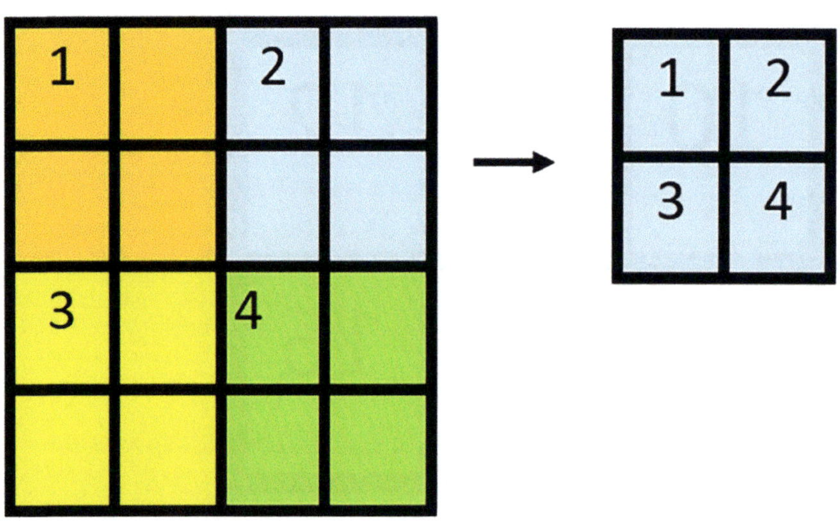

Figure 5.7 Diagram of block scanning pattern

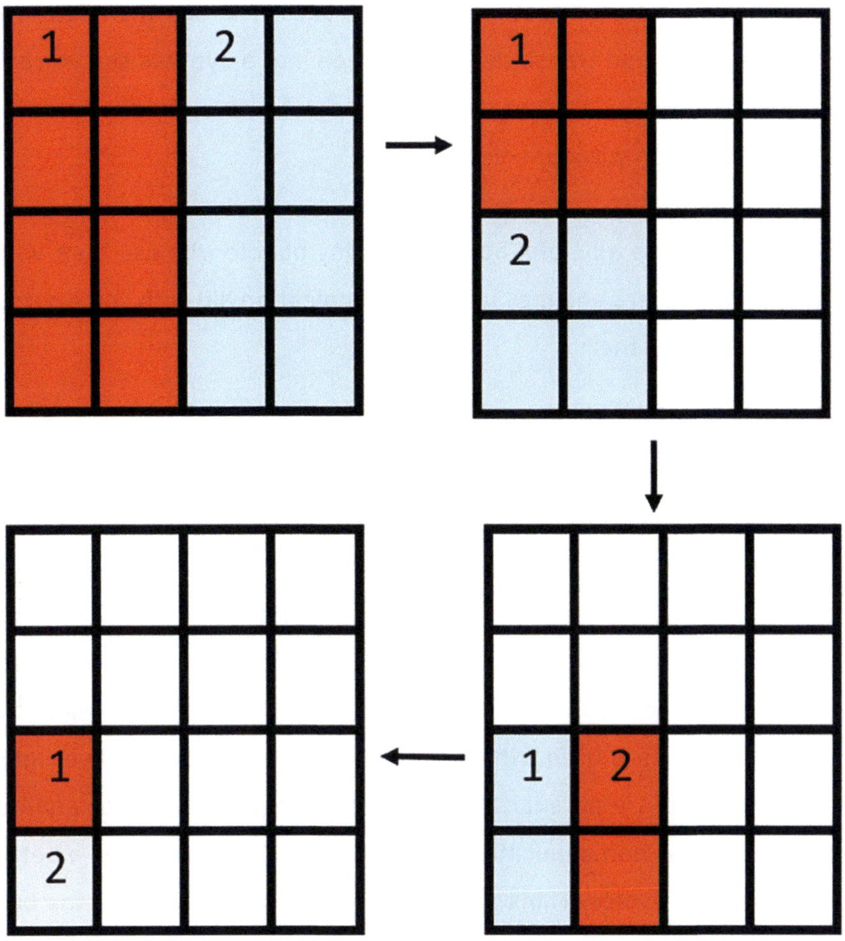

Figure 5.8 Diagram of elimination scanning

Voice input Voice Output Communication Aids

Many people use their own speech with familiar communication partners who are able to understand them. With less familiar communication partners, using Voice Input Voice Output Communication Aids **(VIVOCAs)** is becoming a feasible option as a way to access AAC (Hawley et al., 2012).

VIVOCAs use automatic speech recognition, which is commonly used with smart phones and smart home platforms, to enable those with dysarthric speech to translate their utterances into written text or a synthetic voice. The person records themselves saying words and phrases into the software, which then learns to recognise their individual speech.

Some apps will allow a person to record vocalisations into the app and match them to set words or phrases. The person then speaks to the app on their phone or tablet, which interprets their vocalisation (Voice Input) and plays the associated message (Voice Output).

Other apps, such as Project Relate (Google LLC), use a process similar to voice banking where the user records themselves saying at least 500 phrases. The app then listens to the person speaking (Voice Input) and translates their speech into a synthesised voice on a communication aid (Voice Output). The user can also choose to have the app translate their speech into text on the screen without voice output.

VIVOCA technology is proving to be a helpful option for many people who use their voice with familiar communication partners and may use a communication aid with voice output for less familiar communication partners.

Voice

Choosing a voice

Powered communication aids use either recorded voices (single and multi-message devices) or synthesised voices (computer or tablet communication aids, although these can also usually use recorded voices too). For either option, it is important to consider the person's preference for which voice is used. When recording speech onto a single or multi message communication aid, often a parent, speech and language therapist or another adult will record their voice. If the communication aid user is a child, it might be a better idea to ask a peer to record their voice. Think about the gender too. As always, the best thing to do is to involve the child in choosing whose voice is recorded.

When setting up a communication with a synthesised voice, a prompt is given to choose a voice from a given selection. The range of voices available is increasing, however the choice is currently fairly limited in terms of regional accents. It can be easy to assume which voice a person would prefer and to make that choice on their behalf, however good practice would be to involve the person in the selection of their voice. Avoid making assumptions about age, gender and accent.

AAC software will usually have the option to adjust the pitch and speed of the available voices. This can be a useful consideration when selecting a voice as minor adjustments to these settings can produce a variation on a standard voice that might be preferred by the user. For practitioners working in settings with multiple AAC users, using different voices for each AAC user might be a consideration. This is often not possible if the people arrive in the setting having already chosen their voice, as it would be inappropriate to make someone change their voice just because other users have the same voice. However, when setting up a communication aid for the first time, practitioners may consider the voices already used in their setting. Adjusting the pitch and/or speed of the voice might allow for each voice to be subtly different so each AAC user can easily be identified in a busy, noisy environment such as a classroom. While this is a consideration, an AAC user should always have the final say in the voice that is chosen and not have to change their voice to suit the setting or practitioner. It is common place to have settings where multiple AAC users share identical voices without issue.

For multilingual AAC users, the availability of a synthesised voice in their home language is important. The phonemes used in individual languages differ, and as such the synthesised voice needs to reflect the pronunciation of the spoken language accurately. At present, the availability of synthesised voices in languages other than English is limited and may be restricted to one gender, or an adult voice, which may be inappropriate for the AAC users (Small et al. cited in Pert, 2022).

Voice and message banking

For people whose voice is currently intelligible, they may choose to bank their voice to use on a communication aid in future. For further information around voice banking, **voice repair** and **synthetic voice design**, see chapter seven.

Considerations for autistic AAC users

For AAC users who use echolalia (either internally or externally), being able to record a spoken word or phrase onto their powered communication aid is essential. If the echoed message comes from a television programme, film or video, using the exact clip might be helpful. The echolalia might also come from a family member or someone close to them, such as their mum singing a song. Getting this person to record themselves saying the phrase and adding this to the cell on the communication aid can be important. This is because the intonation, pitch, accent and rate of how the phrase is said can be incredibly meaningful to the autistic person. Using a synthetic voice to say these phrases may not be as helpful. Communication aids may therefore use a mixture of both the synthetic voice and a recorded voice.

Some autistic people may also find voice output (whether recorded or synthetic) too stimulating, and prefer to use a communication aid with no voice output. This might vary across time, environment and situation. On one occasion voice output might be preferred, and at other times the person might want to have no voice output and rely on their communication partner to look at their message on the screen. Practitioners may wish to consider adding a button/cell that turns the voice output on and off and teaching the AAC user how to find this and use it independently.

Organisation

The way in which vocabulary is presented or organised on a communication aid (both paper-based or powered) is often referred to as the organisational method. The words used to describe the organisational methods will vary greatly, including words such as package, language, system and layout (Judge et al., 2020).

The term vocabulary package will be used here to describe a product which has been developed to represent language within a communication aid. The term **organisational method** will be used to describe the way in which these graphic symbols, photographs, letters or written words are arranged within the vocabulary package.

Representing concepts using symbols

The term symbol is often used in reference to a pictorial representation of a concept, either printed on a piece of paper or shown on the screen of a communication aid. Strictly speaking, as symbol is any mode which is used to convey a concept. This might be a gesture, spoken word, written letter, photograph or drawing.

There are several methods used to describe and classify symbols within the literature. Until recently, the most used system was the AAC Model by Lloyd et al., in 1990 and 1992 (cited in Pampoulou and Fuller, 2021). Lloyd et al. saw symbols as being either aided or unaided. Within these two groups, symbols could be static or dynamic, iconic or opaque, and either a set or a system. For a full explanation of these terms, see Pampoulou and Fuller (2021). This classification has recently been challenged by Pampoulou and Fuller (2021) who suggest clarifying symbols using two categories:

1) The design attributes of the symbol(s):
    a) **Physical attributes** refer to the dimensionality of aided symbols (e.g., 3D, 2D, animated, acoustic).
    b) **Design attributes** refer to the type of symbol (e.g., object, pictorial, line drawings, phonemic or phonetic based, alphabet based, vocal).
2) The linguistic characteristics of the symbol(s)

a) **Non-linguistic symbols** do not hold internal logic, being without rules which would allow the user to generate new symbols (e.g., objects, photographs, pointing, vocalisations).
b) **Prelinguistic symbols** hold some element of internal logic that allow some expansion (e.g., Makaton, Widgit).
c) **Linguistic symbols** have internal logic that allows unlimited expansion (e.g., American Sign Language, Blissymbolics, Braille).

Collections of symbols which do not hold internal logic (generative rules), or only a little, might be referred to as **symbol sets**. Collections which do hold internal logic might be referred to as **symbol systems** (Pampoulou and Fuller, 2021).

When we are talking about symbols on communication aids, we are thinking about either graphic symbols or the alphabet/written words. Graphic symbols might be single meaning, representing a single concept, for example a picture of an apple relates to the word "apple".

Multi-meaning symbols or **icons** use word association to change the meaning of a single symbol/icon according to a second graphic symbol which is selected. For example, in Minspeak®, the icon for *bed* can be combined with the icon for *noun* to produce *bed*, or it can be combined to the verb icon to produce *sleep*. This method might also be referred to as **semantic compaction** or **encoding** (Baker, 1994).

Choosing a graphic symbol set or system for someone can often be a complex decision. There might be an established symbol set or system in the person's environment already. Their school or day setting may have other AAC users and adopt a "whole setting" approach, only using one set or system. Sometimes this adoption may spread city- or region-wide. Some AAC vocabularies only present a limited number of options for symbol sets/systems. If the AAC vocabulary takes higher priority than the symbol system/set, then this might be the deciding factor.

A common concern is that switching from one graphic symbol set/system will be confusing for a child. There are several reasons why changing might be considered. Perhaps the person moves from one area to another and their current symbol set/system is not supported in their setting. It could be that a person has trialled one AAC vocabulary for a while but there is consideration about changing to a different one which doesn't support the same symbol set/system. **Motor planning theory** would suggest that the appearance of the symbol set/system is less important than the location of the symbols. Those using a symbol system rather than a set, where internal logic is used to generate vocabulary, may find the change more challenging.

We will now move on to consider how both the alphabet and graphic symbols can be organised on paper and powered communication aids.

Types of displays

AAC displays can be static or dynamic. Static/fixed displays are vocabulary packages using just one page. Some examples include an alphabet chart/board, a core board or a 'Blissymbolics © board (often referred to as a Bliss board or chart).

Paper-based static displays can offer the user a practical AAC solution as they are easily portable and can be laminated to increase the durability and water-resistance. Using waterproof, non-tear paper to print the display, or a matt laminate, will reduce the chance of reflection that is associated with gloss laminates. Powered communication aids might also use static displays, discussed previously in Chapter 4 under *static overlay communication aids*.

Static displays using graphic symbols might be produced around a specific activity, perhaps for short-term use (see Figure 5.9). This could be related to a story book that a class are studying, where graphic symbols of the characters are added to a display, or it might be themed around a national holiday, such as bonfire night in the UK.

Static displays might also be developed using core vocabulary and are often referred to as **core boards**. Core boards are designed not to be used in short-term activities, but instead the vocabulary is selected to be valuable across a range of contexts. They are freely available from most of the communication aid companies, although each companies' version will differ slightly (see Figure 5.11).

Dynamic displays are vocabulary packages where selecting an item navigates the user to a different page. The navigation might occur automatically when the user selects a graphic symbol or word (dynamic active) or when the user selects an operational cell, such as "back", "home" or "more" (Reichle et al., cited in Judge et al., 2020). Dynamic displays might be paper-based or powered.

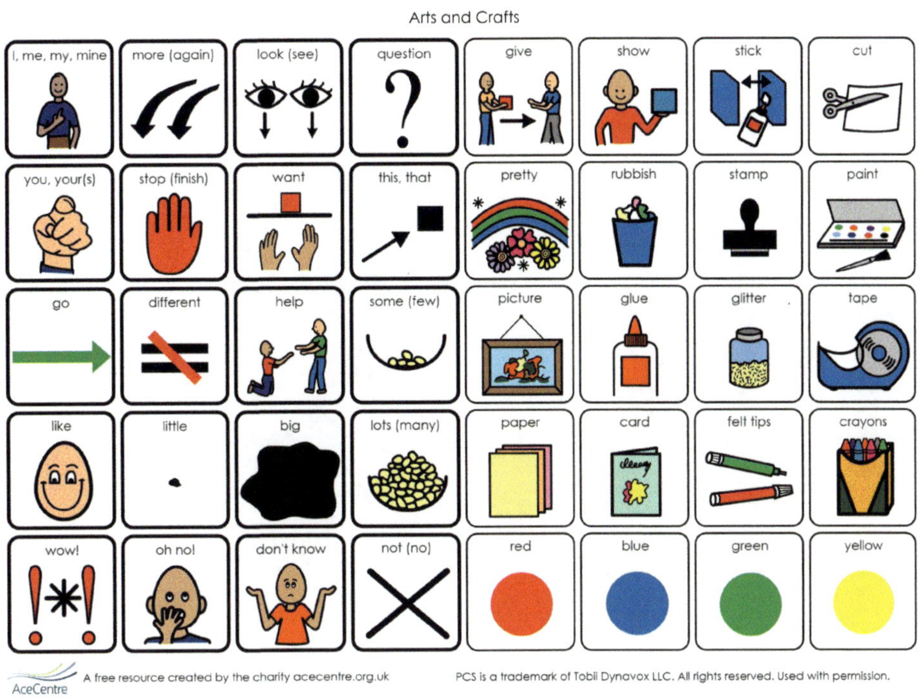

Figure 5.9 An example of an activity-based layout using PCS

Source: produced by Ace Centre. PCS is a trademark of Tobii Dynavox LLC. All rights reserved. Used with permission.

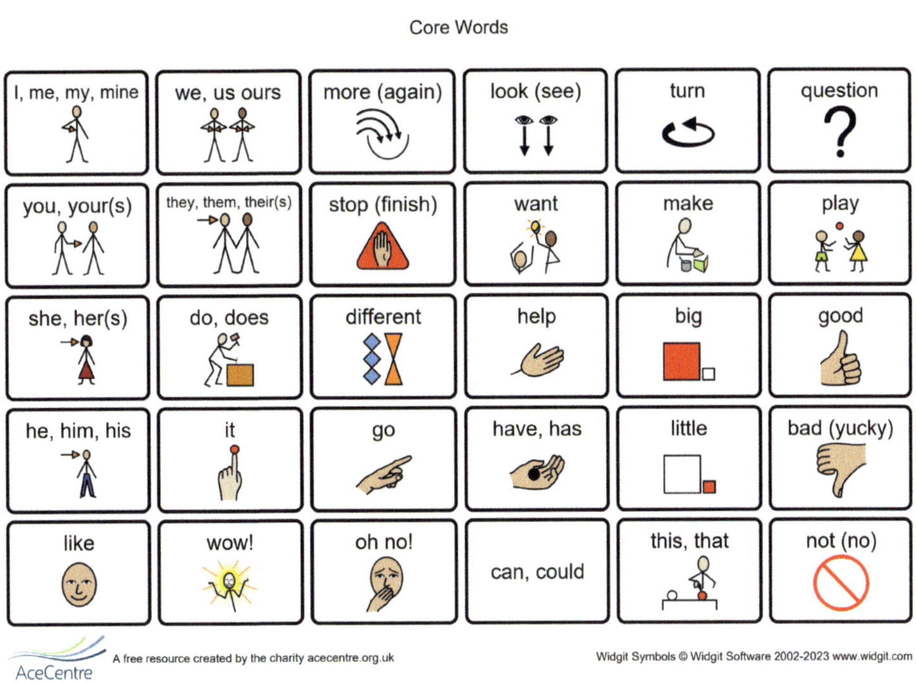

Figure 5.10 An example of a core board using PCS

Source: produced by Ace Centre. PCS is a trademark of Tobii Dynavox LLC. All rights reserved. Used with permission.

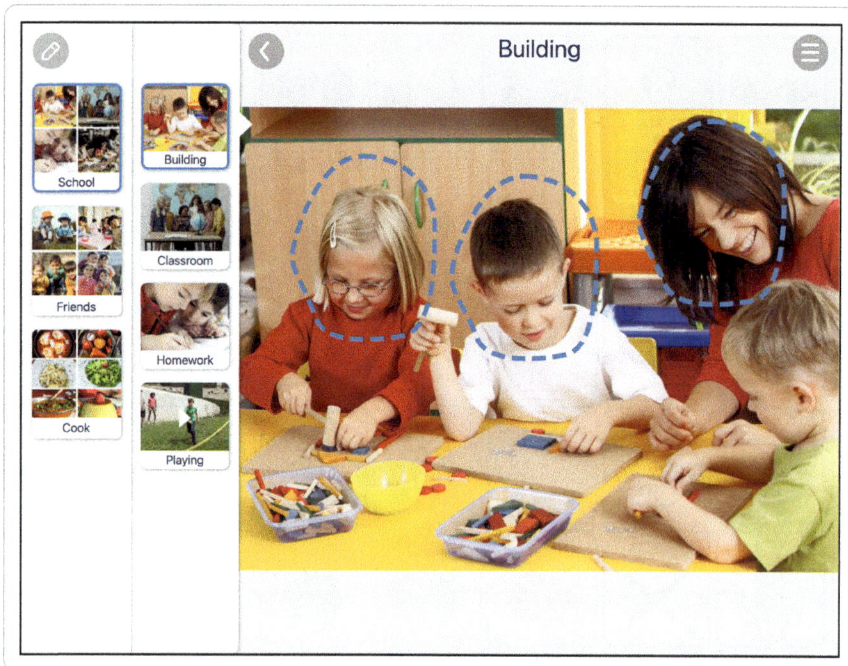

Figure 5.11 A visual scene from the app "Scene & Heard" by Therapy Box

Successful use of a dynamic display requires three specific skills. First, the person needs to understand that items exist within the vocabulary package. Second, they need to know where each item is located within the vocabulary package. Third, the person must learn and remember the navigational route to get to the item (Drager et al., 2003, 2004).

Ways of presenting the vocabulary on a page

Choosing the most appropriate way of representing and organising language for an individual is a complex decision and one which can impact the successful use, or abandonment, of their AAC (Moorcroft, Scarinci and Meyer, 2021).

It's worth noting that most vocabulary packages have been developed using the logic of adults without communication difficulties and differences, and much of the research into organisational methods has used people who are not AAC users (Drager et al., 2003; Fallon, Light and Achenbach, 2003).

Grid-based layouts

Vocabulary packages have historically used a grid-based layout, where items are displayed in rows and columns. The individual items within these girds might be referred to as *cells* or, particularly when displayed on a powered communication aid, *buttons*. The linguistic and cognitive demands of navigating through grid-based layouts have been noted in several studies.

There are vocabulary packages with different stages or levels, often designed with the intention that users will progress from one stage to the next with the development of their language skills. Stages might be labelled according to the number of cells on each page, or simply by a letter or name (Judge et al., 2023a). This option often appeals to practitioners and families as it is seen to be easier than giving a new AAC user too much vocabulary at once, thinking this might overwhelm them. Giving a smaller grid size (with larger cells) might also help people who struggle to access more cells on a page due to physical access needs. Visual processing might also be given as a reason for selecting an AAC vocabulary with fewer items on a page. Some published assessments will test a person's ability to find a target item on pages of increasing numbers of cells. While these are important factors to consider, it is worth thinking ahead and being aware of the pitfalls of changing grid size to allow for language growth. When someone learns where a concept is stored in their AAC vocabulary, they establish motor patterns, which might speed up their access to vocabulary (motor planning or motor patterning). Moving from one grid size to another will interrupt the established motor patterns which is likely to make it harder for the user to find vocabulary (Judge et al., 2023b).

Visual scene displays (VSDs)

The 1980s saw the emergence of visual scene displays (see Figure 5.11) as an alternative way of representing vocabulary (Beukelman et al., 2015; Wallace, Hux and Beukelman, 2010).

A photograph or drawing sets the scene (see Figure 5.11). On powered communication aids, a spoken message is either recorded into the aid, or programmed in via the software. Selecting part of the picture, sometimes called a "hot spot", will produce a word or phrase (Dietz, McKelvey and Beukelman, 2006; O'Neill, Light and Pope, 2018). In other VSDs, the graphic symbols are be positioned next to the photograph or picture, with the message spoken (by the communication partner if the aid is paper-based, or by the powered communication aid). These might be called "hybrid displays" (Beukelman and Mirenda, 2005). VSDs may also be referred to as "schematic scenes" (Wilkinson, Stutzman and Seisler, 2015).

Studies using children without communication difficulties or differences have shown that young children (age 3 and under) are more likely to use a VSD to communicate, especially when photographs and symbols are combined, than a communication aid with only graphic symbols (Drager et al., 2003, 2004; Wilkinson et al., 2015).

The use of VSDs has also been shown to be beneficial for some adult AAC users. The use of photographs to give context to the conversation, along with easier navigation routes compared to grid-based vocabularies, is thought to be beneficial, especially for people with aphasia. This might be because people with aphasia are able to make use of preserved visuo-spatial skills to differentiate between subjects in the photographs, which maintain their relative features such as size and shape. Comparatively, graphic symbols that are presented in a grid layout are of a similar size (e.g., a house is the same size as a car), making them harder to identify (Beukelman, Thiessen and Fager, 2021; Thiessen, Thistle and Brown, 2021).

Personalisation of VSDs has been shown to be important for people with aphasia. Where possible, using photographs of the person themselves, their friends and relatives is beneficial. If this isn't possible, then matching the person's age and gender is helpful (Beukelman, Thiessen and Fager, 2021; Thiessen, Thistle, and Brown, 2021).

VSDs do not pose demands on the AAC user in terms of message formulation, compared to graphic symbol vocabularies with a grid layout and may be a preferred option for both children and adults with a range of communication needs (Thiessen, Thistle, and Brown, 2021).

Photographs can be described as no-context, low-context or high context.

No-context photographs would show the object, person or animal against a white background.

Low-context photographs might have an environment without people or animals, or people and animals in an environment but not interacting with it.

High-contrast photographs include people, objects or animals within an environment and interacting with it.

Studies have looked at the preferences of people with aphasia and people with brain injuries and highlighted the importance of context for these two groups (Beukelman, et al., 2021; Dietz, McKelvey and Beukelman, 2006; Wallace, et al., 2010). It is important to carry out individual assessments within the brain injury population, as response to no-context, low-context and high-context photographs can vary. For people with aphasia, high-context photographs have been shown to be most helpful (Beukelman, Thiessen and Fager 2021; Dietz, McKelvey and Beukelman, 2006). The additional contextual clues and relatedness to the person's own life (by using them and their family and friends, and their own environment) can support understanding.

Ways of organising the pages in the vocabulary package

The method by which the items within a vocabulary package are organised can be described as follows:

- **Taxonomic:** Vocabulary is organised within categories, using a hierarchy e.g., food breakfast items toast.
- **Semantic syntactic:** Vocabulary is organised within linguistic categories e.g., pronouns, nouns, verbs. This also might be referred to as linguistic-based navigation.
- **Schematic:** Vocabulary is organised around an "event schema" e.g., breakfast time.
- **Pragmatic:** Vocabulary is organised according to functions of language e.g., asking a question, requesting, or giving an opinion.
- **Encoded:** Two or more items are sequenced to produce a word or message. This includes the use of colour or numerical encoding (see Figures 5.16 and 5.17) and semantic compaction (Baker, 1994), explained earlier in this chapter.

(Banajee, Dicarlo and Buras Stricklin, 2003; Beukelman et al., 1984; Beukelman and Mirenda, 2005; Drager et al., 2003; Murray and Goldbart, 2016; Webb et al., 2019)

It is tempting to try and fit individual vocabulary packages into one type of organisational method, however, in reality most vocabulary packages use a combination of several organisational methods and might be referred to as hybrid (RCSLT 2024). For example, the **Pragmatic Organisation Dynamic Display (PODD©)** communication system (developed by Gayle Porter in 2007) might be assumed to be a pragmatically organised vocabulary, as the name suggests, however, it makes use of pragmatic *and* semantic organisational methods, along with core and fringe words (Korner, Carter and Stephenson, 2023). Many AAC vocabularies will use a semantic/syntactic layout on the top level, or "home" page, which uses core vocabulary and will then link to taxonomically organised pages (see Figure 5.12).

Taxonomic organisation

Vocabulary items are arranged in a grid layout categorically (topic based), for example, people, food or places. The person selects one of the categories and is directed to a new

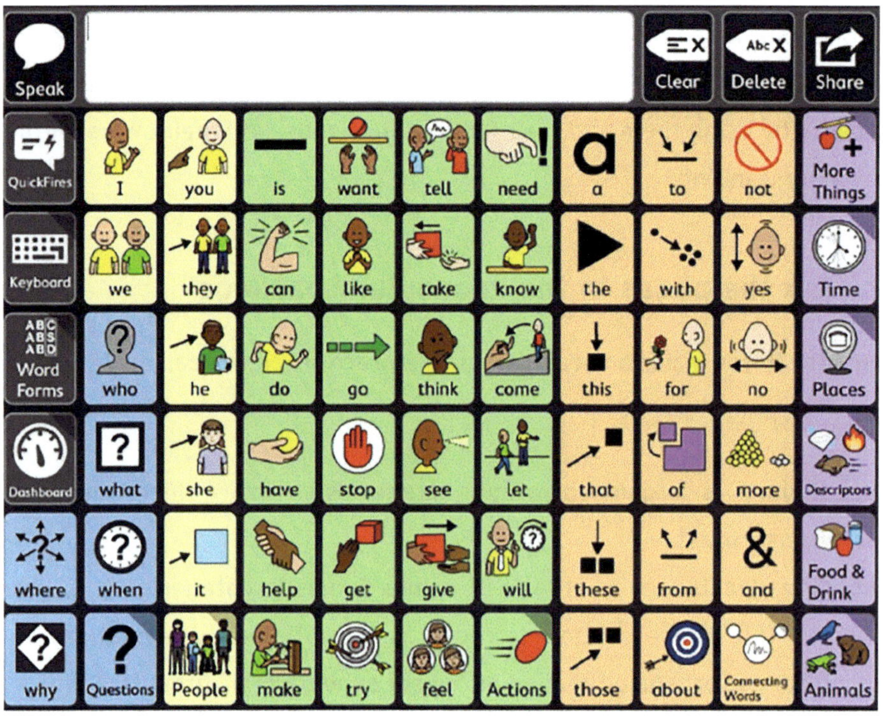

Figure 5.12 An example of a vocabulary combining semantic/syntactic organisation with taxonomic organisation

Source: screenshot taken from Tobii Dynavox Motor Plan vocabulary. PCS is a trademark of Tobii Dynavox LLC.

grid, which may contain further subordinate categories and pages. Selecting "people" might take the person to a page with further categories such as "family"' "school people" and "friends". Selecting one of these subordinate categories will then lead to vocabulary.

Many vocabulary packages use taxonomic organisation; however, this may be a challenge to some people. Younger children (aged three and below) without communication difficulties or differences find both taxonomic and schematic organisation challenging to learn, however, studies have shown that taxonomic layouts were much harder to use compared to visual scene displays. It is suggested that this is likely to be due to the high demands placed on working memory skills by taxonomic organisation. Children's categorisation skills develop at around six to seven years, therefore using taxonomic organisation for young AAC uses has not been recommended (Beukelman and Mirenda, 2005; Fallon, Light and Achenbach, 2003).

The demands of taxonomic organisation have also been considered in relation to people with aphasia, who are likely to find these challenging due to impairments in both working memory and categorisation skills. The navigation through taxonomic layouts might be challenging. The graphic symbol used to represent the subordinate category may not be easily relatable to the page it links to. The challenges of using taxonomic organisation have also been highlighted for people with brain injury (Wallace, Hux and Beukelman, 2010).

Semantic/syntactic organisation

Vocabulary items are grouped according to the parts of language. For example, pronouns, verbs, prepositions. The word groups are often ordered from left to right to facilitate the production of sentences which mirror the spoken language, for example, prepositions, verbs, nouns. Word groups will usually be colour-coded, often using the modified **Fitzgerald Key** (McDonald and Schultz, 1973) or a system developed by Goossens et al. (1994) as shown in Table 5.2 (cited in Beukelman and Mirenda, 2005).

Although most AAC vocabularies will use one of the colour coding systems shown in Table 5.2, there may be additional variation to colour coding. The creators of the app Proloquo, AssistiveWare, opted to group by "word kinds" and consequently chose a different colour coding system. In the development of the Proloquo app, AssistiveWare noted that many words can belong to multiple word groups/kinds. For example, "paint" can be both a noun and a verb (Niemeijer and Sheldon, 2024). This can present a challenge when using colour coding in a semantic/syntactic organisation. Some AAC vocabulary developers may opt to assign a word to only one group, or it may be placed in multiple groups.

Another system for colour coding language, **Colorful Semantics** (Bryan, 2003), is used outside of the field of AAC, to support children with their use of grammar and word order. The

Table 5.2 Two systems for colour coding semantic/syntactic displays

Word group	*Modified Fitzgerald Key*	*Goossens, Crain and Elder*
verbs	green	pink
adverbs	brown	blue
adjectives	blue	blue
nouns	orange	yellow
prepositions	pink	green
negation, emergency words	red	orange
determiners	grey	orange
questions	purple	orange
pronouns	yellow	orange
conjunctions	white	orange

coding used in Colorful Semantics does not match that of the colour coding systems used in most graphic symbol vocabularies. Practitioners will frequently question what to do if a child they are supporting is already using the Colorful Semantics system and AAC is being introduced. There is much support for the use of colour coding to support language development and agreement that consistency of the colour coding is important, however there is no easy solution to the question raised when a child is exposed to two coding systems (Beukelman and Mirenda, 2005; Boster and McCarthy, 2018; Franco et al., 2018). While much graphic symbol software offers the ability to change the colour coding, this is often a laborious task. In the real-world, we are left with the less-than-ideal scenario where a child is exposed to two differing colour-coding systems. Most do seem to manage however.

Labelling word groups using terms such as "prepositions" and "adjectives" is probably not helpful for most AAC users and their families. AAC developers have responded to this by using alternative terms, including "describing words" and "little words". Some companies have opted to remove the word group labels altogether and simply use colour coding to signify each group.

People with aphasia are likely to find semantic syntactic organisation challenging (Beukelman, et al., 2021).

Vocabulary might be grouped in semantically related pairs. For example, "hot" would sit next to "cold" and "loud" would sit alongside "quiet". This is known as semantic association.

Schematic organisation

This method might also be referred to as environmental or activity-based organisation. Words or phrases are grouped according to an activity or place. For example, a grid about breakfast time might include words such as television, iPad, cereal, dog and the names of family members if these are the words associated with the AAC users typical breakfast time. Words are likely to appear across multiple grids. For example, "dog" might appear on the breakfast page, house page and car page.

Pragmatic organisation

Vocabulary items are organised according to their communicative function. For example, asking questions, requesting something or giving information (see Figure 5.13).

People with aphasia are known to have impaired pragmatic skills, such as asking questions and distinguishing conversation openers from conversation closers. The use of colour

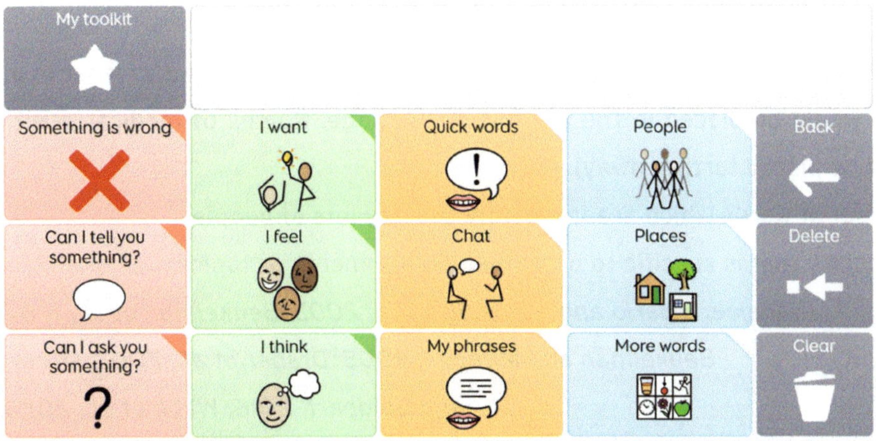

Figure 5.13 An example of a pragmatic graphic symbol vocabulary, taken from *Voco Chat* by Smartbox

coding with pragmatic organisation has been shown to be beneficial for people with aphasia (Beukelman, et al., 2021).

Pragmatic branch starters link to pages of vocabulary and help set the context for the message being communicated. This is said to be helpful for children who cannot rely on gesture or intonation to support their communication (Moorcroft, et al., 2021). Indicating the communicative context of the message being given could be one advantage of pragmatic organisation.

The most well-known graphic symbol vocabulary that uses a pragmatic organisation it the PODD© communication system (Porter, 2007). It important to refer back to an earlier section of this chapter in which we note that the PODD© system actually uses a variety of ways to organise vocabulary. Still, its primary organisational method is pragmatic. Given the popularity of this approach, it is surprising that very few studies have investigated PODD©. Those that have investigated PODD© have focused on the implementation of the **Aided Language Stimulation Approach** using PODD© (see Chapter 6), rather than the organisational method itself (Korner, Carter and Stephenson, 2023). Moorcroft, Scarinci and Meyer (2021) call for further research into the effect of pragmatic branch starters on expressive language.

Ways to organise vocabulary on a page

The method by which vocabulary is organised within individual pages can be described as follows:

- **Alphabetic:** Vocabulary is organised according to the alphabet e.g., "A" words, "B" words etc.
- **Frequency:** Vocabulary is arranged in order, from most frequently used to least (e.g., family names would be placed in the top left of the page. Names of medical practitioner's would be placed further away).
- **Core:** A small set of words which are frequently used by lots of people.
- **Fringe:** Vocabulary that is specific to particular environments or topics.

(Banajee, Dicarlo and Buras Stricklin, 2003; Beukelman et al., 1984; Beukelman and Mirenda, 2005; Drager et al., 2003; Murray and Goldbart, 2016; Webb et al., 2019).

Alphabetic organisation

Vocabulary items are organised according to the first letter of the written word. For example, "animal" and "apple" would be placed together in a folder labelled "A words". This method can be helpful for people who have the ability to quickly recall the initial letter of a written word.

Frequency organisation

Vocabulary is organised according to frequency of use. Concepts which are likely to be used more often are placed in the top row of a page. The subsequent rows have vocabulary which is less likely to be used. Frequency organisation is most likely to be used to organise a list of fringe vocabulary, for example, on a page of drinks the person's favourite drinks would be on the top row and their least preferred drinks on the bottom row.

Core vocabulary

Many popular graphic symbol vocabularies use a combination of core and fringe vocabulary. Core vocabulary are words/concepts which occur most frequently in a language. Core vocabulary allows AAC users to communicate across a range of contexts and build novel messages. Examples of core words include; more, stop, help, me, you, go, want, like.

The core vocabulary lists used to develop popular graphic symbol vocabularies are based on the spoken and written language samples of older children and adults, both with and without communication differences or difficulties (Laubscher and Light, 2020; Robinson, 2023b). In studies that suggest core vocabulary lists, samples were taken across a range of contexts, such as classrooms, work places and semi-structured interviews. It is worth considering how the context of the language sampling will likely impact the resulting frequency of words. Laubscher and Light (2020) and Robinson (2023b) have highlighted the need for further research that samples the language of younger children and also people with communication needs and differences, including AAC users, when creating core vocabulary lists.

Fringe vocabulary

Fringe vocabulary is a word/concept that is additional to core vocabulary, and often a noun. For example, food items, people's names, animals, TV shows, book titles, places. Fringe vocabulary will often be highly personal.

Many graphic symbol vocabularies use a combination of a core vocabulary page and many fringe vocabulary pages. This would be a combination of a semantic/syntactic and a taxonomic organisation. The suggestion is that AAC users will combine core and fringe vocabulary to create novel messages e.g., "want car".

Ways to organise vocabularies that use the alphabet

The organisation or layout of the letters and/or words can make accessing the display more efficient. The alphabet can be organised in different ways:

QWERTY layout*:* where the letters are organised in the same way as a computer keyboard, starting in the top left with the letters QWERTY. This layout can be helpful for people who are familiar with using a computer keyboard and if they are still able to use their fingers to access the display, as motor planning skills will likely allow for efficient spelling.

ABC layout: where the letters are organised alphabetically. This might be helpful for a person who isn't familiar with a QWERTY layout.

Frequency layout: where the letters are organised according to how frequently they occur in the language spoken by the AAC user. The more frequently occurring letters would be placed in the top left. This layout can increase efficiency and reduce fatigue if accessing the display is effortful (see Figure 5.14).

Whole word/phrase layout: where frequently used words or phrases are written in full. This method can be helpful if the person is not able to spell words reliably, but can read whole words. This might be the case for people with emerging or developing literacy, or for

Space	E	A	R	D	U
T	O	I	L	G	V
N	S	F	Y	X	.
H	C	P	K	J	,
M	B	W	Q	Z	?
Delete letter	Start again				

AceCentre

To use: Ensure you have an agreed signal for "yes" and ideally "no". Hold the chart so it can be seen easily. Speak aloud and / or point to the first item on each row. When the person indicates yes, offer each letter / command / message in turn along that row (including the first option) until they indicate "yes". Speak aloud the letter, command or message they have selected and then restart the process. If you speak aloud something that is incorrect, they can indicate "no" or go on to select 'Delete letter' or 'Start again' on the chart. It is easier to keep track of the conversation if you write down letters as they are selected. If the person is happy for you to predict what word they might be spelling, check you have guessed correctly before moving on to the next word or phrase. Before putting the chart down, always ask if they have more to say. Visit www.acecentre.org.uk for more information.

Figure 5.14 An example of a frequency letter layout
Source: produced by Ace Centre with permission.

people with a brain injury. Whole word layouts can also be beneficial for people who find accessing AAC effortful as one selection can communicate a whole word instead of spelling out each letter. Sometimes, keyboards will be included alongside the words for times when novel words need to be spelled (see Figure 5.15). Static displays might use a combination of whole words, letters and graphic symbols.

Encoding

Colours or numbers are used to "code" the letters or words, often to support access and increase efficiency. The person first selects the block or area of the page that contains their chosen letter or word (the target). Then, they will select the colour or number on the page that corresponds to their target within that area. For example, in Figure 5.16, if wanting to select the "S", the person would first select the grey box because it includes the letter "S" and then select the blue box because the "S" is blue. Encoded layouts can be an efficient way to formulate a message if pointing is effortful or not possible. Figure 5.17 shows numerical encoding.

Abbreviation expansion: where there is an agreed code between the AAC user and communication partner. The AAC user selects a combination of letters which are an abbreviation of a longer phrase. Figure 5.18 shows that if the letters "HRU" were selected, this would communicate the message "how are you?"

qu	w	e	r	t	y	u	i	o	p	0	1	2	3
a	s	d	f	g	h	j	k	l	DELETE	4	5	6	7
SPACE	z	x	c	v	b	n	m	.	?	8	9	£	:
about	above	after	afternoon	all	an	and	as	ask	at	bad	best	better	big
by	bye	call	can	can't	children	come	day	do	don't	down	early	evening	feel
few	find	first	from	get	give	go	good	great	have	he	hello	help	her
high	his	home	homework	house	in	inside	into	it	know	large	last	late	leave
left	like	little	long	look	love	make	man	many	more	morning	my	next	night
not	number	of	old	on	or	other	outside	over	own	part	person	place	play
right	same	say	school	see	she	small	some	stop	tell	that	the	there	they
thing	this	time	under	up	use	way	want	week	will	with	woman	work	worse
worst	year	you							please	thank you	yes	no	don't know

Chart developed by the charity acecentre.org.uk. Visit website for more resources.

Figure 5.15 An example of a whole word layout with a keyboard, "QWERTY chart with useful words for a child"

Source: produced by Ace Centre with permission.

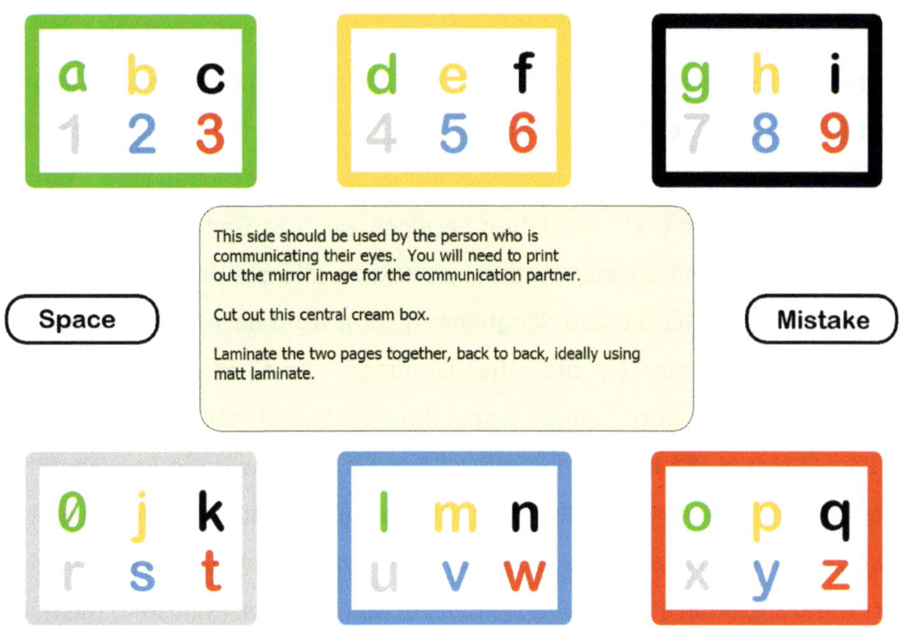

Figure 5.16 An example of colour encoding with the alphabet

Source: taken from "Alphabet Chart Pack" produced by Ace Centre.

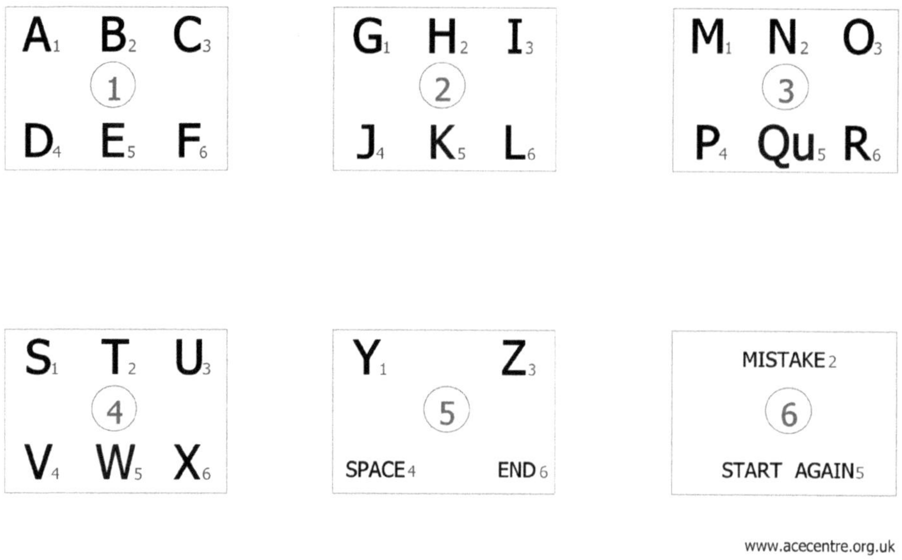

Figure 5.17 An example of numerical encoding
Source: taken from "number encoded ABC you can point to" produced by Ace Centre.

Language

Culturally appropriate vocabulary

Communication aids which use graphic symbols must provide both culturally appropriate vocabulary and graphic symbols (Huer, 2000). The majority of graphic symbol vocabularies are developed in English. Over recent years, increasing attention has been drawn to the need for properly developed graphic symbol vocabularies in other languages. There is sometimes an assumption made that translation services, such as Google Translate, are adequate ways of converting an English vocabulary package into another language. This is not a reliable way of producing a useful language system from an AAC user, as many English words do not translate directly into other languages. Small et al.(in Pert, 2022) give the example of the English word "more" translating as "additional", "extra" or "further", which would not match the intended linguistic function of "more" in English. While the developers of graphic symbol vocabularies are beginning to respond to this need, an alternative solution might be to use a native speaker of the home language, or a paid interpreter, to support the translation of a graphic symbol vocabulary from English to the home language. An important consideration is that written translation and verbal translation services are often separate, and practitioners may need to seek support from both, at an increased cost compared to using one service that offers both written and verbal translation (Small et al., in Pert, 2022).

I use Letter Codes so I can be quicker at saying my message.

Keep this list pinned up on the wall so we can all see it.

Add new Letter Codes to this list when I ask you to.

IP → I'm in pain (please get my pain scale)
TA → tell me about...
HRU → how are you?
PC → please call...
RW → remember when...

Figure 5.18 An example of abbreviation expansion
Source: taken from "Abbreviation Expansions" produced by Ace Centre.

Some people will need a full graphic symbol vocabulary in their home language, whereas others may only need a small selection of words or phrases. It can take significantly longer to develop graphic symbol vocabularies in languages other than English (Royal College of Speech and Language Therapists, 2022). Giving the person a few words, phrases or pages of vocabulary to begin with and gradually building on this can be a better solution than withholding a communication aid from them whilst a full vocabulary is developed (Sadiku et al., in Pert, 2022).

When considering culturally appropriate vocabulary, we may initially be drawn to the words associated with the food, clothing, religion and leisure activities of that culture. It is perhaps fairly obvious that this fringe vocabulary will need to be personalised to reflect the lived experiences of the individual AAC user. It may be less obvious to consider the need to vary the core vocabulary across cultural contexts. Western graphic symbol vocabularies use language samples of English-speaking children and adults to determine a list of high frequency words (Laubscher and Light, 2020). These are the words that can be used flexibly across communicative contexts to convey a wide range of meaning. In English, these include words such as more, stop, go, help, me, you, want and like. The core vocabulary of languages other than English may be quite different (Small et al., in Pert, 2022). Draffan et al. (2015) gathered data from existing graphic symbol vocabularies in use by Arabic speaking AAC users, along with other vocabulary sources such as reading lists. These lists were analysed to produce a core vocabulary for Arabic, which was then compared to English core vocabulary lists. The Arabic core vocabulary contained a number of nouns (e.g., ball, banana and chair) which in English graphic symbol vocabularies would be considered fringe vocabulary. The Arabic core vocabulary list did also share similarities with the English core vocabulary lists, in that both feature conjunctions and prepositions.

Culturally appropriate graphic symbols

Iconicity refers to how similar the graphic symbol and referent are (how well the graphic symbol represents the concept or word). The higher the iconicity of a graphic symbol, the easier it is to recognise and learn (Kang et al, 2019). The ease of learning to understand and use graphic symbols for each individual is also related to their life experiences, cultural background and time exposed to the graphic symbols (Beukelman and Mirenda, 1998, cited in Heur, 2000).

Studies by Heur (2000) and Kang et al. (2019) have looked at the perceptions of different graphic symbol sets across groups of adults with different cultural backgrounds. In both studies, participants were asked to rate each graphic symbol in terms of iconicity and the results showed that each person's cultural background and life experiences influenced their perceptions. This can have a significant impact when choosing a graphic symbol vocabulary, as an AAC practitioner may select a graphic symbol set, or individual symbols, which are perceived very differently by the AAC user. For this reason, the AAC user and/or their family should always be involved in selecting a graphic symbols system, and/or individual graphic symbols for concepts.

Some concepts will be consistent across the world, yet the graphic symbol will need to differ. Pampoulou and Fuller (2020) give the example of the concept "post box", which will be red in the UK, yellow in Cyprus and blue in the USA. Consequently, the graphic symbol will need variation depending on the country.

It is important to consider the cultural variation across one country. Pampoulou and Fuller (2020) give the example of Texas in the USA, which has a large Hispanic population. Large countries, such as Pakistan which borders the countries of Iran, Afghanistan, China and India, will have significant cultural variation. The food eaten in the northeast will be influenced by Chinese culture, the food eaten in the east and southeast will have Indian influences. Consequently, the graphic symbol chosen to represent the concept of food may need to differ. The fringe vocabulary within the category of food will look very different for AAC users in one area of Pakistan compared to another (Butt, 2023).

Graphic symbols may also differ in the concepts associated with them. For example, the symbol of "thumbs up" can have both positive and negative associations depending on the cultural context (Pampoulou and Fuller, 2020).

The representation of people in graphic symbol vocabularies must be culturally appropriate, in terms of skin tone and clothing. Most of the commonly available graphic symbol sets now offer a choice of skin tone.

Resources

Global Symbols aims to make culturally appropriate graphic symbol sets freely available. Developers of graphic symbol sets can publish their graphic symbols for free on the Global Symbols website. The symbol sets can also be downloaded for free and the website offers the ability to create graphic symbol boards to print:

https://globalsymbols.com/?locale=en

Most graphic symbol vocabularies will have the written word above or below the graphic symbol. It is important to be aware that some languages may not have a standardised written form.

For people who use the alphabet on their AAC (text to speech), there are also considerations for those using language other than English. The keyboard on the communication aid (whether paper based or powered) will need to reflect the characters used in the person's home language. Some text to speech app developers now offers the function to switch between two keyboards, word prediction and voices.

Message banking might be a helpful tool when establishing text to speech communication aids for people using languages other than English.

Summary

This chapter has considered some of the choices we make when providing someone with AAC. This includes the hardware (the communication aid), the access method, any mounting requirements and the software. Within the software, we have choices to make about the voice, language and vocabulary organisation.

Decisions made when providing a person with AAC can influence the likelihood of them using it, or abandoning it. There are a range of ways to display and organise vocabulary on a communication aid and a variety of terms which are used interchangeably. We might use a grid layout, or a visual scene display. There are features of both which will suit different groups of people and careful assessment is required.

Letters, written words and phrases can be organised in a number of ways to support efficient access to the alphabet. Graphic symbol vocabularies can be organised using a range of methods and often several methods will be used within one vocabulary package. The term "robust AAC" is widely used to describe the key features all AAC systems (which might be one mode of AAC or a collection) should have.

References

AssistiveWare. (accessed 31 October 2023). 4 things every AAC system needs. www.assistiveware.com/learn-aac/select-a-balanced-aac-system.

Baker, B. R. (1994). Semantic Compaction: An Approach to a Formal Definition. Proceedings of 6th Annual European Minspeak Conference.

Banajee, M., Dicarlo, C. and Buras Stricklin, S. (2003). Core vocabulary determination for toddlers. *Augmentative and Alternative Communication*, 19(2), 67–73. https://doi.org/10.1080/0743461031000112034.

Beukelman, D., Yorkston, K. M., Poblete, M. and Naranjo, C. (1984). Frequency of word occurrence in communication samples produced by adult communication aid users. *Journal of Speech and Hearing Disorders*, 49, 360–367.

Beukelman, D., Mirenda, P. (1998). Augmentative and alternative communication: Management of severe communication disorders in children and adults (2nd ed.). Baltimore: Paul H. Brookes.

Beukelman, D. and Mirenda, P. (2005). *Augmentative & Alternative Communication*. Paul H Brooks Publishing.

Beukelman, D. R., Hux, K., Dietz, A., McKelvey, M. and Weissling, K. (2015). Using visual scene displays as communication support options for people with chronic, severe aphasia: A summary of AAC research and future research directions. *Augmentative and Alternative Communication*, 31(3), 234–245. https://doi.org/10.3109/07434618.2015.1052152.

Beukelman, D. R., Thiessen, A. and Fager, S. K. (2021). Personalization of visual scene displays: Preliminary investigations of adults with aphasia, typical females across the age span, and young adult males and females. *Topics in Language Disorders*, 41(3), E1–E11. https://doi.org/10.1097/TLD.0000000000000256.

Boster, J. B. and McCarthy, J. W. (2018). Designing augmentative and alternative communication applications: The results of focus groups with speech-language pathologists and parents of children with autism spectrum disorder. *Disability and Rehabilitation: Assistive Technology*, 13(4), 353–365. https://doi.org/10.1080/17483107.2017.1324526.

Bryan, A. (2003). Colourful semantics: Thematic role therapy. In S. Chiat, J. Law and J. Marshall (eds) *Language Disorders in Children and Adults* (1st ed., pp. 143–161). Wiley. https://doi.org/10.1002/9780470699157.ch10.

Butt, A. L. (2023, September 11). Development of Culturally Appropriate Urdu core Vocabulary Symbols for AAC Users. Communication Matters Conference, Leeds, United Kingdom. https://eu.eventscloud.com/website/9795/programme/.

Demasco, P. W. & McCoy, K. F. (1992), Generating text from compressed input: an intelligent interface for people with severe motor impairments, Communications of the ACM, v.35, n.5.

Dietz, A., McKelvey, M. and Beukelman, D. R. (2006). Visual scene displays (VSD): New AAC interfaces for persons with aphasia. *Perspectives on Augmentative and Alternative Communication*, 15(1), 13–17. https://doi.org/10.1044/aac15.1.13.

Draffan, E. A., Wald, M., Halabi, N., Sabia, O., Zaghouani, W., Kadous, A., Idris, A., Zeinoun, N., Banes, D. and Lawand, D. (2015). Generating acceptable Arabic Core Vocabularies and Symbols for AAC users. 6th Workshop on Speech and Language Processing for Assistive Technologies (pp. 91–96).

Drager, K. D. R., Light, J. C., Speltz, J. C., Fallon, K. A. and Jeffries, L. Z. (2003). The performance of typically developing 2½-year-olds on dynamic display AAC technologies with different system layouts and language organizations. *Journal of Speech, Language, and Hearing Research*, 46(2), 298–312. https://doi.org/10.1044/1092-4388(2003/024).

Drager, K. D. R., Light, J. C., Carlson, R., D'Silva, K., Larsson, B., Pitkin, L. and Stopper, G. (2004). Learning of dynamic display AAC technologies by typically developing 3-year-olds: Effect of different layouts and menu approaches. *Journal of Speech, Language, and Hearing Research*, 47(5), 1133–1148. https://doi.org/10.1044/1092-4388(2004/084).

Fallon, K., Light, J. and Achenbach, A. (2003). The semantic organization patterns of young children: implications for Augmentative and Alternative Communication. *Augmentative and Alternative Communication*, 19(2), 74–85. https://doi.org/10.1080/0743461031000112061.

Franco, N., Silva, E., Lima, R. and Fidalgo, R. (2018). Towards a Reference Architecture for Augmentative and Alternative Communication Systems. 1073. https://doi.org/10.5753/cbie.sbie.2018.1073.

Goossens', C., Crain, S., Elder, P. (1992). Engineering the Preschool Environment for Interactive, Synbolic Communication. Birmingham, AL: Southeast Augmentative Communication Conference Publications.

Hawley, M. and Cunningham, S., Green, P., Enderby, P., Palmer, R., Sehgal, S. and O'Neill, P. (2012). A voice-input voice-output communication aid for people with severe speech impairment. IEEE transactions on neural systems and rehabilitation engineering: A publication of the IEEE Engineering in Medicine and Biology Society. 21. 10.1109/TNSRE.2012.2209678.

Huer, Mary Blake. (2000). Examining Perceptions of Graphic Symbols Across Cultures: Preliminary Study of the Impact of Culture/Ethnicity. *AAC Augmentative and Alternative Communication*, 16, 180–185.

Judge, S., Nasr, N. and Hawley, M. (2018). A user-centred approach exploring the potential of a novel EMG switch for control of assistive technology. In P. Cudd and L de Witte (eds) *Harnessing the Power of Technology to Improve Lives* (Vol. 242, pp. 381–384). IOS Press.

Judge, S., Randall, N., Goldbart, J., Lynch, Y., Moulam, L., Meredith, S. and Murray, J. (2020). The language and communication attributes of graphic symbol communication aids – A systematic review and narrative synthesis. *Disability and Rehabilitation: Assistive Technology*, 15(6), 652-662. https://doi.org/10.1080/17483107.2019.1604828.

Judge, S., Murray, J., Lynch, Y., Meredith, S., Moulam, L., Randall, N., Whittle, H. and Goldbart, J. (2023a). Attributes of communication aids as described by those supporting children and young people with AAC. *International Journal of Language & Communication Disorders*, 58(3), 910–928. https://doi.org/10.1111/1460-6984.12833.

Judge, S., Murray, J., Lynch, Y., Meredith, S., Moulam, L., Randall, N., Whittle, H. and Goldbart, J. (2023b). Attributes of communication aids as described by those supporting children and young people with AAC. *International Journal of Language & Communication Disorders*, 58(3), 910–928. https://doi.org/10.1111/1460-6984.12833.

Kang, R., Kim, Y. T. and Yeon, S. J. (2019). Cultural differences on the recognition of social word AAC graphic symbols between Korean and American undergraduate students. *Communication Sciences & Disorders*, 24(1), 71–86. https://doi.org/10.12963/csd.18542.

Korner, H., Carter, M. and Stephenson, J. (2023). Coaching parents of young children with complex communication needs to implement aided language stimulation using pragmatic organisation dynamic display communication books. *International Journal of Disability, Development and Education*, 1–18. https://doi.org/10.1080/1034912X.2023.2166676.

Laubscher, E. and Light, J. (2020). Core vocabulary lists for young children and considerations for early language development: A narrative review. *Augmentative and Alternative Communication*, 36(1), 43–53. https://doi.org/10.1080/07434618.2020.1737964.

McDonald, E. T. and Schultz, A. R. (1973). Communication boards for cerebral-palsied children. *Journal of Speech and Hearing Disorders*, 38(1), 73–88. https://doi.org/10.1044/jshd.3801.73.

Moorcroft, A., Scarinci, N. and Meyer, C. (2021). "I've had a love-hate, I mean mostly hate relationship with these PODD books": Parent perceptions of how they and their child contributed to AAC rejection and abandonment. *Disability and Rehabilitation: Assistive Technology*, 16(1), 72–82. https://doi.org/10.1080/17483107.2019.1632944.

Murray, J. and Goldbart, J. (2016). Operational demannds and representational forms. In J. Murray and M. M. Smith (eds) *The Silent Partner? Language, Interaction and Aided Communication* (pp. 35–64). J & R Press Ltd.

Niemeijer, D. and Sheldon, E. (21 October 2024). How Is the Proloquo Vocabulary Organized? Assistiveware Blog.

O'Neill, T., Light, J. and Pope, L. (2018). Effects of interventions that include aided Augmentative and Alternative Communication input on the communication of individuals with complex communication needs: A meta-analysis. *Journal of Speech, Language, and Hearing Research*, 61(7), 1743–1765. https://doi.org/10.1044/2018_JSLHR-L-17-0132.

Pampoulou, E. and Fuller, D. R. (2021). Introduction of a new AAC symbol classification system: The multidimensional quaternary symbol continuum (MQSC). *Journal of Enabling Technologies*, 15(4), 252–267. https://doi.org/10.1108/JET-04-2021-0024.

Pert, S. (2022). *Working with Children Experiencing Speech and Language Disorders in a Bilingual Context: A Home Language Approach* (1st ed.). Routledge. https://doi.org/10.4324/9781003125563.

Porter, G. (2007). Pragmatic Organisation Dynamic Display (PODD) communication books: Direct access templates. Melbourne: Cerebral Palsy Education Centre.

RCSLT (2024). Augmentative and alternative communication (AAC) – Guidance. Royal College of Speech and Language Therapists. www.rcslt.org/members/clinical-guidance/augmentative-and-alternative-communication/augmentative-and-alternative-communication-guidance/#:~:text=This%20guidance%20aims%20to%20support%20RCSLT%20members%20to

,be%20achieved%20by%20using%20evidence-informed%20practice%2C%20which %20includes%3A.

Robinson, H. (2023a) The Positive AAC Framework [Poster presentation], Communication Matters Conference, 12 September, 2023.

Robinson, H. (2023b). My Research internship: Investigating the core vocabularies provided to people who use symbol communication aids. *Communication Matters Journal*, 37(1), 9–11.

Sadiku, L., Small, K., Martin., (2022). Augmentative and alternative communication. In Pert, S. (2022). *Working with Children Experiencing Speech and Language Disorders in a Bilingual Context: A Home Language Approach* (1st ed., (pp. 181-196). Routledge. https://doi .org /10 .4324/9781003125563.

Thiessen, A., Thistle, J. and Brown, J. (2021). Clinical and research perspectives on visual scene displays. *American Journal of Speech-Language Pathology*, 30(3), 1134–1156. https://doi.org/10 .1044/2021_AJSLP-20-00212.

Todman, J., Alm, N., Higginbotham, J. & File, P. (2008), "Whole utterance approaches in AAC", Augmentative and Alternative Communication, v. 24, n.3.

Wallace, S. E., Hux, K. and Beukelman, D. R. (2010). Navigation of a dynamic screen AAC interface by survivors of severe traumatic brain injury. *Augmentative and Alternative Communication*, 26(4), 242–254. https://doi.org/10.3109/07434618.2010.521895.

Webb, E. J. D., Lynch, Y., Meads, D., Judge, S., Randall, N., Goldbart, J., Meredith, S., Moulam, L., Hess, S. and Murray, J. (2019). Finding the best fit: Examining the decision-making of augmentative and alternative communication professionals in the UK using a discrete choice experiment. *BMJ Open*, 9(11), e030274. https://doi.org/10.1136/bmjopen-2019-030274.

Wilkinson, K. M., Stutzman, A. and Seisler, A. (2015). N400 brain responses to spoken phrases paired with photographs of scenes: Implications for visual scene displays in AAC systems. *Augmentative and Alternative Communication*, 31(1), 51–62. https://doi.org/10.3109/07434618.2014.965342.

Zangari, C. (2021, December). PrAACtical Questions. "What Does a Robust AAC System Look Like?" *PrAACtical AAC*. https://praacticalaac.org/praactical/praactical-questions-what-does-a-robust -aac-system-look-like/.

6

PRACTICE AND PLAY

Helen Robinson

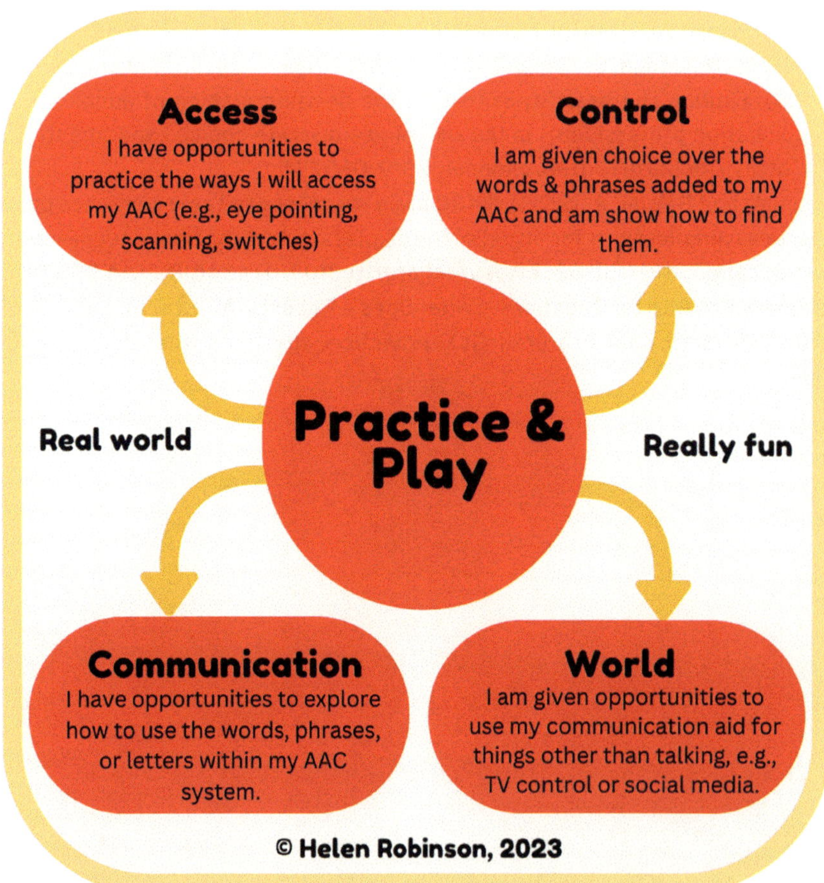

Figure 6.1 The AAC Practice and Play strand from The Positive AAC Framework
Source: Robinson (2023).

- Access
  Practicing switch scanning
  Practicing partner-assisted scanning
  Practicing eye pointing

DOI: 10.4324/9781003412311-8

- Partner-assisted scanning (page 1 of 3)

  How to use partner-assisted scanning:
- Partner-assisted scanning (page 2 of 3)
- Partner-assisted scanning (page 3 of 3)
- Control

  Language for self-advocacy

  Language for regulation

  Language which is personal

  Language to describe

  Language which is taboo

  Language to use in different places
- Choosing language for AAC (page 1 of 2)
- Choosing language for AAC (page 2 of 2)
- Communication

  Aided AAC input

  AAC prompt hierarchies

  Communication temptations

  How do we model well?

  Modelling AAC for analytical language learning style

  Modelling AAC for gestalt language learning style

  Modelling for people with acquired communication difficulties

  Modelling without expectation

  What do we do when someone doesn't like us touching their AAC?

  AAC and literacy
- Tips for supporting emergent readers and writers who use AAC (page 1 of 2)

  Shared reading

  Shared writing
- Tips for supporting emergent readers and writers who use AAC (page 2 of 2)

  Alphabet and phonological awareness

  Independent writing with access to the full alphabet

  Self-directed reading
- Tips for supporting literacy for people who use AAC (page 1 of 2)

  Reading comprehension
- Tips for supporting literacy for people who use AAC (page 2 of 2)

  Word study

  Writing

  Self-directed reading

Once an individual has been provided with AAC, next comes the task of supporting them to learn to use it. This chapter explores the "practice and play" strand from The Positive AAC Framework, shown in Figure 6.1 (Robinson, 2023). We will consider how someone might be supported to practice using their access method(s), how they might be involved on choosing and setting up the words on their AAC and how they might practice using them. Finally, we will consider other ways that AAC can give a person control of their world by exploring computer access, social media, gaming and environmental controls.

Access

Chapter 5 considered the different ways a person might access or control their AAC. Here, we will look at how we can provide opportunities to practice scanning and eye pointing, which can benefit from a more structured pathway.

Practicing switch scanning

Learning to use a switch to access a powered communication aid takes physical and cognitive effort. This can be especially challenging for young children (McCarthy et al., 2006). Following an assessment to select an appropriate switch (or switches), it's necessary to support the person to learn to use their switch(es) to access technology. For some, beginning with communication software might be too challenging, because failing at communicating due to your access method is frustrating, and they will need opportunities to practice using their switch(es) in other ways.

Several teaching frameworks are available to support the development of switch skills. These are shown is Table 6.1. Note that The Seven Stages of Switch Development (Jiao Ltd. Switch Heroes – Jiao) is based on the other two packages (Bean, 2011; Burkhart, 2018). While all three use subtle differences in their stages and descriptions, essentially they each outline a similar process: exploring using one switch, adding in a second switch, moving and choosing, errorless learning and independent switch scanning. While these frameworks all include practicing with a second switch, it's important to notes that not everyone will have the physical or cognitive abilities to be able to control two switches. These frameworks can still be used by those who use one switch.

Table 6.1 A comparison of three switch skills programmes

Stage	*Switch Progression Learning Journeys Road Map, Inclusive Technology (Bean, 2011)*	*Stepping Stones to Switch Access Linda Burkhart (2018)*	*The Seven Stages of Switch Development (Jiao Ltd. Switch Heroes - Jiao)*
1	Experiential learning	Single switch: cause and effect	Learning by experience: single switch
2	Making something happen	Single switch: multiple locations and multiple functions	Making something happen: single switch
3	Playing with two switches	Two switches: two functions	Playing with two switches. Making two things happen
4	Choosing independently	Learning to two switch step scan	Two switches, one activity
5	Introducing formal scanning (always right)	Two switch step scanning: Failure free learning with feedback	Switch scanning, failure free
6	I can use one or two switches to make choices	Two switch step scan to a target	Switch scanning, finding the right one
7		Practice for increasing accuracy with two switch step scanning	Independent functional switch use
8		Switch automaticity: reducing time for success and demonstrating knowledge	

Key points when practicing switch use

- Avoid prompting the person to "press the switch" as it encourages compliance. Independent exploration is best.
- Let the person know what's happening when they press the switch, e.g., "You made the music start".
- Consider starting with fewer items to scan through and add in more as the person gains confidence.

Ideas for activities to practice switch use

- Switch toys
- Environmental control items (see "World" later in this chapter)
- Computer games and apps
- Specialist switch scanning software
- Accessing YouTube
- Online puzzle games

Strategies to make switch scanning easier

Setting up switch scanning often involves more than selecting an appropriate switch or switches. We can make adjustments to the scanning patterns, how items are highlighted, how items are selected and the feedback that is given (McCarthy et al., 2006). Each piece of software will have differences in the options available for adjusting the switch scanning settings. See the resource *Switch access to technology: A comprehensive guide* (Judge and Colven, 2006) for a detailed explanation of the adjustments which can be made.

Practicing partner-assisted scanning

Using partner-assisted scanning (sometimes referred to as listener mediated scanning) takes practice. The handouts in this chapter should help to explain the process to those who are supporting someone to use this method to access paper-based AAC. Partner-assisted scanning might also be used with objects or for people with visual impairment, who won't rely on the visual resources, but will purely listen to your voice. There are two key factors when introducing this method:

Consistency: Start in the same place each time, and scan through the items in the same order. This will help the AAC user to predict what's next. Agree the strategy the AAC user will use to confirm their selection, how you will check you've understood their choice, and what you will both do if the AAC user's response isn't clear.

Honesty: As a communication partner, it's important we admit if we have missed or misunderstood the AAC user's response. Be clear and let them know what you think they have communicated, rather than assuming. Offer them a choice to try again, or move on.

Practicing eye pointing

Clarke et al. (2022) explored looking behaviours in children with cerebral palsy. They describe a developmental progression of looking skills as shown in Figure 6.2. This scale can support us to observe how a person is using their looking behaviours and consequently if and when they might be able to use these skills to access paper or powered AAC. People will need to be using the skills at all stages (5–1) before they can use their vision to make choices for communication. Learning to use eye-gaze technology for young children is challenging. Learning to understand that their eye movements directly affect what is happening on the screen can take time. Software and activities alone may not be sufficient to teach this skill and children benefit from additional adult instruction (Griffiths, Clarke and Swettenham, 2023). Practice should be consistent, ongoing and embedded throughout the day (Karlsson et al., 2021).

Further resources

- Eye-gaze control technology for people with cerebral palsy: 2021 Clinical Guidelines www.ausacpdm.org.au/resources/eye-gaze-control-technology-for-people-with-cerebral-palsy-2021-clinical-guidelines/
- Look 2 Talk is a package which outlines the steps to developing eye pointing as an access method for paper-based AAC. Available from: https://acecentre.org.uk/resources/look2talk

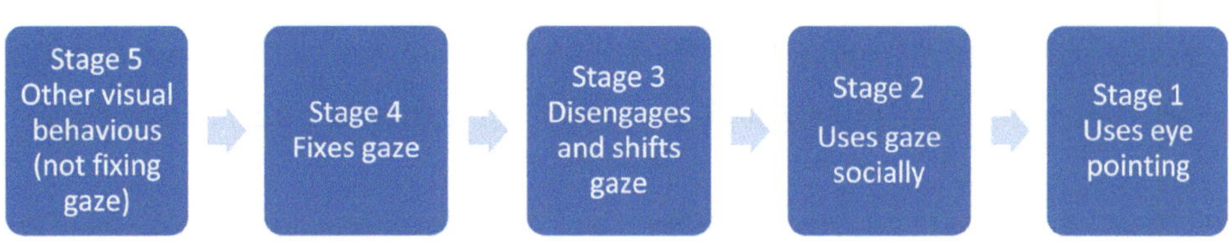

Figure 6.2 Summary of the stages of the UCL eye pointing classification scale
Source: Clarke et al. (2022).

Partner-assisted scanning (page 1 of 3)

Augmentative and Alternative Communication (AAC) can help people to express themselves. This might be through objects, an alphabet or symbol chart or a communication book. If an AAC user finds it difficult to point, we can help them make a choice using partner-assisted scanning.

The communication partner ether reads aloud the options, points to them, or both together. The AAC user listens and/or watches as the options are given to them. The AAC user then indicates "yes" in some way when their choice is reached. There are different patterns you can use to scan the items; these are shown on page 2 and 3. Scanning one item at a time can be simpler, but also slow. Other pattens, like row-column scanning, can be quicker but take time for the AAC user to learn.

How to use partner-assisted scanning:

- Choose your scanning patten (see pages 2 and 3).
- Make sure you know how the AAC user will tell you "yes". This might be through words, sounds, facial expressions or body movements. They might use several ways.
- When starting out, it can be helpful to explain to the AAC user what you are going to do. For example, "I'm going to point to the pictures and say the words. You listen and tell me 'yes' when I get to the right one".
- If the AAC user is unfamiliar with the objects, photos, symbols, or words, they might need you to tell them each one (e.g., shoe, coat, hat, shirt, socks). If they are familiar and have good vision, they may manage with you either just pointing or saying "this one?".
- If the AAC user indicates a clear choice, you should confirm this, either by repeating the word, or saying "you want" and then the word e.g., "you want shoes".
- If their response is unclear, tell them what you're noticing. For example, "I think I saw you smile. I think that means yes". You might also say "You made a noise then. I think you're telling me this one".
- If you scan through all the items and haven't observed a clear "yes", tell the AAC user explain you will give them the options again. If you are still unsure, offer them a choice to repeat another time. It's also helpful to give them the option of "it's none of these".

Be honest and be consistent. If you haven't understood their response, apologise and offer to try again. Always scan through the options in the same way, each time.

Partner-assisted scanning (page 2 of 3)

There are the different patterns we can use when scanning through choices:

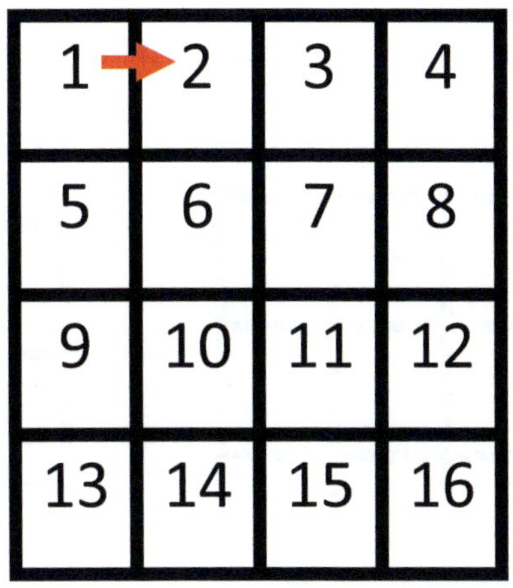

Single item scanning: The communication partner moves through the items one at a time, starting from the top left and moving across the row, then to the left of the second row, across, to the left of the third row and so on.

Row-column scanning: The communication partner points to each row in turn. When the AAC user makes a selection, the scanning continues along the row (one column at a time). The AAC user then makes a second selection to confirm their choice. This method requires the user to be familiar with the items on their communication aid but can be a useful method for increasing speed.

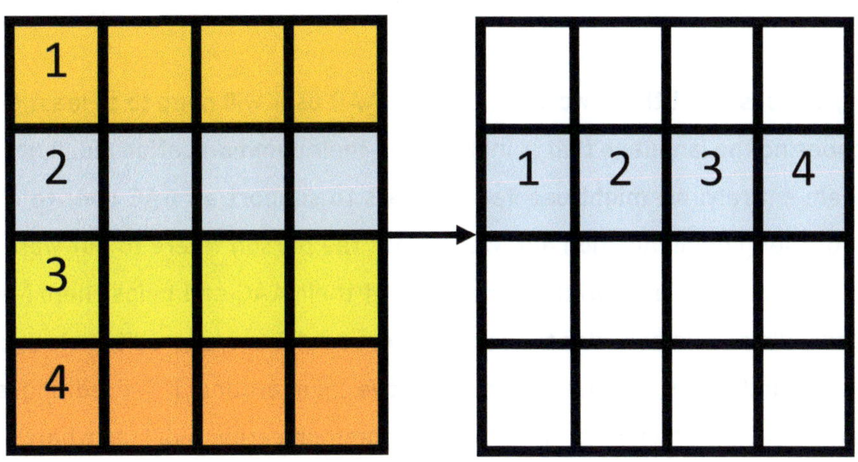

Partner-assisted scanning (page 3 of 3)

Block scanning: The items on the page are grouped into blocks. The communication partner, points to one block at a time. The AAC user makes a selection and then the scanning continues, item by item, within the chosen block. The AAC user makes a second selection to confirm their chosen item.

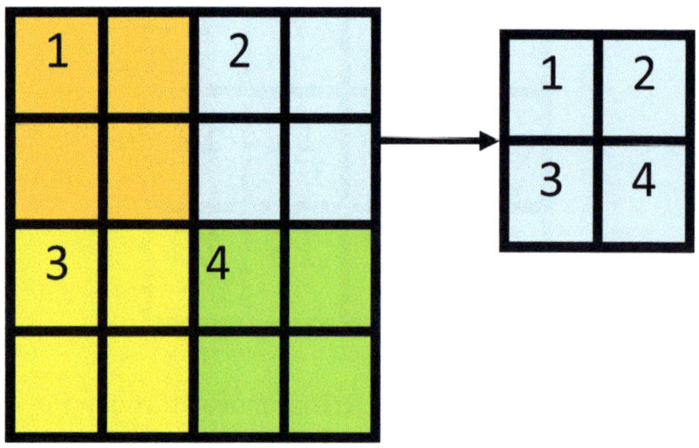

Control

Often, the language provided to people on AAC systems is chosen for them. It is of course challenging to ask an AAC user what words they feel they need before they are capable of using AAC. Those with degenerative conditions will likely have more control in planning ahead regarding the language they might need (even literate AAC users are likely to rely on some pre-stored phrases).

It is usually the case that those working with the AAC user will need to at least guide them towards choosing the language that is included on their communication aid, if not selecting without them entirely. We might use Talking Mats to support an AAC user to choose the language for their communication aid. We can ask the person where to put words on their communication aid. This encourages ownership of their AAC and helps them learn where to find words. We should consider teaching powered AAC users to edit their vocabularies themselves; to add words, remove words and move them around. If self-editing is not possible, adding a button which says "put it on my communication aid!" (or whatever word is used to describe the AAC) can be a very simple but effective tool. If the AAC user hears someone saying a word or phrase, they can select this to let someone know that they need this on their communication aid.

Disabled people are likely to routinely rely on others to do things for them, or to them. Ensuring we give them as much control as possible over their aided language is something we should strive for. This might mean having difficult conversations with the person themselves or their families. It might mean that assessments take longer as we find ways to include them in conversations.

The following is a guide to help us think about the kind of language to consider when setting up a communication aid (whether that is paper or power-based).

Language for self-advocacy

Self-advocacy is about being able to put across your own views, opinions and interests. This includes words and phrases that allow the person to:

- Refuse, reject and protest (e.g., stop it, don't do that, no!)
- Give negative opinions (e.g., I don't like you, I hate it, it's awful)
- Speak up for their rights (e.g., my opinion counts, you didn't ask me, it's in my care plan).

Disabled people are more likely to comply or agree with the demands and requests of others and therefore it is especially important to provide language which allows them to protect against verbal, physical, financial or sexual abuse (Chandler, Russell and Maras, 2019).

Language for regulation

Some people, especially autistic people, might need language to self-regulate (more on this in chapter nine). This can include:

- Words and phrases tell people when they feel overwhelmed (e.g., it's too loud, there are too many people, the light hurts my eyes).
- Words and phrases to rate their levels of regulation (e.g., I'm calm, I'm anxious, I'm not okay).
- Words and phrases to ask for what they need (e.g., I need my blanket, I need a quiet space).

Language which is personal

While core words can be helpful for lots of AAC users, fringe vocabulary which relates to their own interests is important. But beyond this, it's important to ask family members about any particular words or phrases that are used at home. It's common for families to have "inside jokes" and particular ways of saying things. Couples will often have words and phrases which is known only between the two of them. This could include:

- Scripts for daily routines (e.g., night-night, sweet dreams, see you in the morning!)
- Made up words and phrases.
- Family phrases that have perhaps been passed down through generations.
- Alternative names for each other.

Language to describe

Graphic symbol systems may provide people with a basic range of adjectives and adverbs, but some people might need a much wider range of concepts in order to fully articulate their thoughts and feelings. AAC users who rely on graphic symbols may compose poetry, songs or stories. They may find that the vocabularies available to them fail to offer all they need.

Language which is taboo

A fairly common concern for those working with AAC, it whether to provide words and phrases which can be seen as taboo: things that people don't like to talk about, or words which might offend. This can include words and phrases relating to:

- Sex, sexuality and gender (including contraception and sexual health)
- Illness, death and suicide
- Disability
- Race, culture and religion
- Violence and war
- Politics
- Swear words
- Body parts
- Bodily functions (including menstruation and pregnancy)
- Finances (discussing earnings, savings, debt etc.)
- Relationships (break-ups, dating, marriage and divorce)

Adding these words can often be a concern for parents. It's also not uncommon as practitioners to encounter families who hold strong opinions about particular topics and do not want their child to have access to these words. In these situations, we can consider how we would approach these issues if the person were not an AAC user. We must also consider the risk associated with not providing this language, especially where it might prevent the person from advocating for their rights or disclosing abuse.

We might offer advice to parents in the same way we would if their child was speaking. That is, children must learn when and where it is appropriate to use certain words and as adults, we have a responsibility to both provide them with the words and learn how to moderate their use. As practitioners, we need to keep returning to these conversations and have our own personal responsibility to advocate for the AAC user to the right to access the language they might need (Battye, 2023).

Language to use in different places

Code switching is a common part of communication, where we vary the words that we use (or the language we speak) depending on the people we are with or the context we are in. We all know the words to use at work and the words we can get away with using at home! AAC users also might need to do this, especially adults who have intimate relationships with another/others.

We can provide separate pages for them to go to (e.g., family words), or we might decide to set up two profiles (if they are using powered AAC). The AAC user could then switch between "public" and "private profile". However, this presents a risk of words being updated on one profile and not on the other, if we are not careful the AAC user can end up getting lost between two sets of language! (Beukelman and Mirenda, 2005).

Choosing language for AAC (page 1 of 2)

Augmentative and Alternative Communication (AAC) can help people to express themselves. This might be through a paper symbol book, or software with symbols on a computer that speaks (a communication aid).

When we are setting up AAC for someone, it's important to add words and phrases that are going to be helpful, exiting and powerful. Please use this form to tell us about the language you feel is important to include.

Important topics (please use a separate page to list words/phrases to include on each topic page)	
Family names (Please include any 'nicknames' or 'pet names' that might be used for each person too)	
Pets' names	
Friend's names and other important people e.g., neighbours, carers	
Family phrases or sayings	
Made up words or "silly" words using in your family	

Choosing language for AAC (page 2 of 2)

It is important that AAC users have the language they need to talk about the things which matter to them. Sometimes, the things they might want to talk about can make others feel uncomfortable, just like people who use speech. Rather than avoid these topics, it's helpful for us to discuss what language is appropriate to include and what we are less comfortable including. This form should help you to consider what you feel is or isn't appropriate to include. Please place a tick in the box to tell us if your thoughts about each topic.

TOPIC	Examples	I think this topic should be included	I'd like to discuss this more before deciding	I definitely don't want this topic included	Not now, but maybe in the future
Money	Bank, finance, bankrupt, debt				
Sex and gender	Male, female, transgender, intersex, non-binary				
Sexuality	Gay, lesbian, pansexual, condom				
Swear words	C**p, s**t, f**k				
Illness and death	Dying, poorly, funeral, suicide				
Violence and war	Guns, stab bomb, murder				
Body parts	Penis, breasts				
Bodily functions	Poo, period, vomit, tampon				
Relationships	Dating, divorce, marriage				

Communication

How we provide people with opportunities to learn to use their AAC systems is an important topic. Often, we focus our efforts on the assessment and choosing what to provide, then give less attention to how we are going to support the person to use AAC.

As within many areas of speech and language therapy practice, support might take the form of direct or indirect strategies. Direct support strategies tend to be more instructional and planned, often working one-to-one with the person away from their daily activities. Conversely, indirect strategies focus on embedding the AAC into the environment.

Some direct teaching might be helpful, particularly when learning how to access and operate powered communication aids. Indirect or environmental strategies have been shown to be most effective in supporting AAC use (Clendon and Anderson, 2016; Da Fonte and Boesch, 2018).

Aided AAC input

Modelling has long been used as an effective way to support skill development, not just within AAC but more broadly within speech and language therapy. We learn by observing and experiencing others doing it. There are a number of terms which might be used to describe this approach when applied to AAC, such as **Aided Language Modelling** or **Aided Language Stimulation.**

O'Neill, Light and Pope (2018) provide a summary of commonly used terminology and highlight five differing approaches, describing how they each differ and overlap. Some might focus on environmental supports, where are others are more directive. Most of us working with AAC will be unaware of the details of these specific approaches and their individual variation. In practice, when we use the terms Aided Language Stimulation or Aided Language Modelling, we are generally using these terms to talk about how we demonstrate (model) the AAC strategies that that we are hoping the individual might use.

O'Neill, Light and Pope (2018) aim to avoid confusion over the specific approaches by using the term "aided AAC input". Their meta-analysis of aided AAC input approaches concluded "there is evidence to support the use of partner aided AAC input to enhance a wide range of communication outcomes for individuals who use AAC of various ages, diagnoses, and language abilities" (O'Neill et al., 2018, p. 1762). Aided language input has repeatedly shown to be an effective approach in supporting AAC use throughout the literature (Clendon and Anderson, 2016).

The benefits of aided language input include:

- The communication partner becomes familiar with the aided communication method.
- The interaction is slowed down, allowing more time for the AAC user to process language.

AAC prompt hierarchies

The use of prompting to support AAC use has been widely used over the past decade to support aided AAC input. Several versions of AAC prompt hierarchies have been published, with the original credit being given to the Rocky Bay Positive AACtion resource (Langley, 2023). Rachael Langley based her 2015 version on the Rocky Bay prompt hierarchy, as follows:

- Expectant pause
- Indirect nonverbal prompt
- Indirect verbal prompt
- Request a response
- Gestural cue
- Partial verbal prompt
- Direct model
- Physical assistance.

(Langley, 2023)

Another version of the prompt hierarchy followed in 2016, "the Adapted AAC Prompt Hierarchy" by Kate Ahern (2016). This version situated Aided Language Stimulation as an umbrella above the prompting strategies of expectant pause, indirect visual cues and direct visual cues. In Kate's blog post (Ahern, 2016), she discusses the need to remove direct verbal prompting from other versions of the hierarchy, stating that

> telling a child what to "say" with their talker isn't a cue or prompt. It is a command and usually it is testing. When we equate communication with testing we lose out on what drives communication (and humanity, when it comes down to it) – an inherent desire to connect with another person.
>
> *(Ahern, 2016).*

Kate also warned of the dangers of using physical prompting; taking the person's hand and making them touch the communication aid. This disrespects a persons' body autonomy and teaches them that others have the right to touch them without consent, manipulate their body and force them to communicate.

Despite Kate Ahern's clear warning of the dangers of hand-over-hand prompting, this practice has continued over the past decade. Da Fonte and Boesch (2018) provide an image of an AAC prompt hierarchy which includes full and partial physical prompting and advocate for its use within their description of prompting practices, also known as "errorless learning" stating "prompting provides the student with the support needed to reduce incorrect responds as the student acquires new skills" (Da Fonte and Boesch, 2018, p. 251). Other literature prescribes a variety of graduated prompt fading techniques, often including the use of hand-over-hand prompting (Beukelman and Mirenda, 2005). Biederman et al. (1998) investigated the use of prompting in children with developmental disabilities and found that, while often used, hand-over-hand prompting to be less effective at teaching skills compared to verbal modelling and advocated for it not to be used.

In 2023, Rachel Langley discussed her original intentions behind the AAC Prompt Hierarchy, stating that it was only ever intended as a means to describe the behaviours being observed in classrooms and that she always saw the behaviours higher up the scale as "bad" (Langley, 2023). Her intention was for the hierarchy to serve as a tool for practitioners to identify and call out harmful practice. Instead, the hierarchy was used by many to prescribe how we *should* prompt. Rachel has recently updated the AAC Prompt Hierarchy, which encourages us to consider four health habits:

- Thoughtful pauses
- Expressing interest with body language
- Observing and commenting
- Modelling without expectation

We are discouraged from modelling "so they copy you" and prompting "to make them say it" (Langley, 2023).

Kate Ahern has also revised her Adapted AAC Prompt Hierarchy (Ahern, 2023). In her blog post, Kate emphasises the need to place Aided Language Stimulation as an "umbrella under which all other intervention occurs" and highlights the importance of AAC and communication always being a "choice" (Ahern, 2023). Kate discusses the wishes of many parents and practitioners asking for interventions which are not compliance based, which, along with AAC prompt hierarchies, have dominated AAC interventions for many years (Ahern, 2023).

Communication temptations

Communication temptations have been widely used throughout Speech and Language Therapy, and beyond, as means of supporting the development of communication skills. Communication temptation strategies include the following:

Sabotage: Situations are manipulated or "sabotaged" by the communication partner in order to encourage use of wither a particular word or communication skill. For example; not providing the glue during a craft activity so the AAC user has to ask for "help" or question where the glue is.

Crumbs: The communication partner gives a tiny amount of something highly desired by the person, so they are more likely to ask for more. This might be literally crumbs of food, by breaking a cookie into small pieces or offering one raisin at a time, or it could be something like holding onto all the jigsaw puzzle pieces and only offering one at a time.

Getting things wrong: The communication partner purposefully forgets to do something, or reacts in an unexpected way during a familiar activity.

Challenging: The communication partner sets up a situation that they know the AAC user cannot succeed in independently, so that they will need to ask for support.

These strategies will be labelled in many different ways in practice and in the literature. Da Fonte and Boesch (2018) describe such strategies as "Non-directive Naturalistic Teaching Strategies" (p. 248). Collectively, they are often known as "communication temptations". These have historically been used as a means of creating opportunities for communication, aligned with the *Means, Reasons and Opportunities model* (Money, 1997). They are often highly effective strategies which will be successful in eliciting communication from the individual. However, as discussion regarding the use of prompting has shown, we are now beginning to understand the harm that these strategies may have caused. Communication temptations might appear as being "natural", but if we consider whether we would use these as part of typical interactions with people who do not have communication differences, we begin to see otherwise. Current practice is moving towards an approach of modelling without expectation.

How do we model well?

There are some important differences, and challenges, when modelling language using AAC compared to modelling only speech (for people who don't need AAC). Modelling aided language brings additional challenges. First, AAC users are likely to have a larger receptive-expressive gap, so we are faced with the choice of modelling language at their level of understanding, or at their level of expression. Second, the communication partner is likely to be unfamiliar with the aided language system, impacting the speed at which they can model language. If they are too slow, the person might lose interest and the interaction will be lost. Third, the AAC user is faced with the challenge of listening and watching two forms of input; they are hearing the spoken word while hearing (and watching) the aided langue output.

Modelling AAC for analytical language learning style

People who are learning language through a predominantly analytical style will acquire words in isolation and then add them together, before mastering the grammar and morphology.

When we model spoken language to children who are also using speech, we are aiming to model language which is one step ahead of their current ability. The child's receptive language level will be at a similar level to their expressive language (e.g., they are understanding two key words, and using two-word phrases). We therefore provide a model that is slightly higher than this (e.g., three-word phrases). There is much debate in the literature as to whether we should model the appropriate grammar while reducing the utterance length (e.g., the dog is chasing the ball) or whether we should reduce both the utterance length and simplify the grammar (e.g., dog chase ball). While there is no clear answer, the general agreement is that it's helpful to simplify the utterance while preserving the grammar (Clendon and Anderson, 2016).

When modelling with AAC, most of us tend to give a spoken model with the appropriate grammar, but model a telegrammatic version on the communication aid. For example, if AAC user is beginning to use two-word phrases, we might say "it's time to get your coat on" and model on the communication aid "COAT – ON" (Clendon and Anderson, 2016).

Modelling AAC for gestalt language learning style

People who might be learning language predominantly through gestalt language learning style may be assigning meaning to a chunk of language, which might be a single word or a phrase. Over time, they may then break down (mitigate) these chunks into smaller chunks, then single words, and then go onto build up these single words and acquire grammar and morphology (see Chapter 5) (Blanc, Blackwell and Elias, 2023).

When modelling AAC for people who are non-speaking or minimally speaking, we have to make a best guess at the gestalts to add onto their AAC. As discussed in Chapter 5, this might be a phrase from a favourite film or TV advert, or a line from a song. We provide gestalts which we feel will be motivating for the person. Once the person begins to use the gestalts that we have provided them with, we then provide mitigations of these phrases, while keeping the full gestalt available (we don't remove the original gestalts). For example:

"hey! where'd you go" could be broken down into "Hey!" and "you go"

"up up and away!" could be broken down into "up up" and "and away"

We can then model combining gestalts to make new phrases, for example:

"up up + you go" or "and away + you go"

Alongside modelling gestalts, we can model core words and fringe vocabulary (see Chapter 5). Research into modelling AAC for gestalt language processors is lacking and currently we are learning through our experiences.

Modelling for people with acquired communication difficulties

Much advice so far in this chapter and within the literature focuses on modelling language for children who are emerging AAC users. Advice around supporting this population tends to centre around communication partner training, which is covered in Chapter 7. This is not to say that modelling isn't part of this, which it very much should be. Rather than viewing modelling in terms of developmental stages, modelling for adults with acquired communication difficulties will be centred around contexts and scenarios. For example, practicing using AAC to order a drink in a café, or how to explain discomfort and request assistance. Some adults may wish to explore their AAC system independently and learn through exploration, but others may still benefit from a communication partner modelling use of their AAC system and the features of "good" modelling will still apply to this population.

Modelling without expectation

When supporting people to model using AAC, we must be aware that some may find it difficult to identify what language to model. Practitioners, in particular speech and language therapists, can take this skill for granted. It's important that people working with the AAC users are given clear explanation (and models!) of how to model key words. Practitioners might have a tendency to make modelling seem easy, and fail to realise the challenges of actually doing it in real-life situations (Moorcroft, Scarinci and Meyer, 2021).

As we reconsider our use of prompting and communication temptations, we must consider how this might look. A helpful way to frame this is rather than *creating* (engineering) communication opportunities through strategies like sabotage and crumbs, we *look* for them in natural interactions.

This doesn't mean we can't plan ahead, especially as the communication partners gain confidence in using the AAC. Thinking about the person's interests is a good starting point, making sure these words (or phrases) are on their AAC. We then model these words, in natural situations, without any expectation that the person with use the AAC themselves.

Observing the person and considering what they would say if they used spoken words in a particular situation can be a helpful strategy, then put these words (or phrases) onto their communion aid (and model them!).

Consider the language that the person can already communicate through other strategies (which might be spoken words, gestures, or vocalisations). It's helpful to also model these on their AAC, but it's important not to ask them to use their AAC instead of their current methods. It's up to the person if they choose to use AAC instead of or as well as these strategies.

What do we do when someone doesn't like us touching their AAC?

Some people can become upset if their communication partner attempts to model language using their AAC. This tends to be people who are able to access, hold and carry their AAC around with them. Asking permission to use their AAC might result in the person becoming distressed. In these situations, it's important to recognise and accept the person's right to refuse access to their AAC. If a second version of their AAC is available, the communication partner can model using this. However, if they are using a powered communication aid, resources might be limited and it won't be possible to use a second communication aid. In this scenario, we can make a paper version of their powered system and use that to model. This doesn't necessarily mean reproducing the whole vocabulary package in paper form, but perhaps printing out a few key pages. In some situations, we need to accept that modelling isn't possible and that the person is going to learn to use their AAC through independent exploration.

Key points

- Modelling with AAC is different to modelling only with spoken language.
- Attending to two forms of input can be challenging for the AAC user.
- For people learning mostly through analytical language processing, model the appropriate grammar when speaking, but model key words on their AAC.
- For people learning mostly through gestalt language processing, model whole phrases, alongside core and fringe words.
- Provide clear examples of how to model to those who will be doing it.
- Model without expectation.
- We must respect that some people will not allow us to access their AAC for modelling.

AAC and literacy

Literacy development is an important part of participation in society, providing opportunities for education, employment and relationships (via the use of texting, email and social media) (Ahlgrim-Delzell et al., 2016; Caron, Light and McNaughton, 2020; Light and McNaughton, 2020).

AAC users are often not given opportunities to develop literacy skills (Light and McNaughton, 2020; Sturm, Erickson and Yoder, 2002). Light and McNaughton (2020) highlight that "it has been estimated that up to 90% of individuals who rely on AAC enter adulthood without acquiring functional literacy skills, severely restricting their communication, their educational and vocational outcomes, and their overall quality of life" (p. 428).

Learning literacy utilises both whole word/sight reading, where words are memorised as a whole and decoded, which uses phonological awareness to "sound out" each letter (Barker, Saunders and Brady, 2012; Mandak, Light and Boyle, 2018). Studies investigating teaching literacy to people with communication difficulties and differences tend to focus on the teaching of sight words, and not phonics. It is often assumed that teaching whole word reading is easier. While many of us do use whole word reading, without the ability to decode text phonetically, we will be limited to only reading and writing the words we have been explicitly taught (Ahlgrim-Delzell et al., 2016). Studies have shown that people with communication difficulties and differences, including those with learning disabilities, can learn to read phonetically (Ahlgrim-Delzell et al., 2016; Light and McNaughton, 2020).

Learning to read requires skills across several areas:

- Phonological processing (linking sounds to letter and vice versa)
- Orthographic processing (identifying letters and letter patterns)

- Context processing (experiences and world knowledge to allow understanding of text or to give meaning to text)
- Meaning processing (combining phonological, orthographic and contextual understanding to derive meaning from text, or give meaning to text).

(Adams, 1994, cited in Light and McNaughton, 2020)

Learning to read will be more challenging for AAC users, due to both the characteristics of the individual and their environment.

Individual characteristics include: motor impairments, speech impairments, sensory impairments, working memory difficulties, language impairments, cognitive impairments and real-world experiences.

Environmental factors include: the literacy experiences available, the duration and consistency of literacy teaching, the quality of the literacy teaching and the beliefs of those supporting literacy about the person's potential (Light and McNaughton, 2020; Koppenhaver, 2000; Sturm et al., 2002).

Koppenhaver (2000) acknowledges the additional challenges to literacy learning faced by AAC users, but cautions against assuming that these challenges mean that well-used literacy approaches with non-AAC users should not be implemented. Traditional methods are still applicable to this population, but with some adaptations.

In their book *Comprehensive Literacy for All: Teaching Students with Significant Disabilities to Read and Write*, Erickson and Koppenhaver (2020) break down literacy learning into emergent and conventional. People who cannot yet identify most of the letters of the alphabet, most of the time, do not engage with shared reading and do not understand that print has meaning should begin with emergent reading activities. Those that have achieved these criteria can progress to conventional literacy teaching.

Emergent literacy teaching includes:

- Shared reading
- Shared writing
- Alphabet and phonological awareness
- Independent writing with access to the full alphabet
- Self-directed reading

Conventional literacy teaching includes:

- Reading comprehension
- Word study
- Writing
- Self-directed reading.

(Summarised from Erickson and Koppenhaver, 2020, p. 201)

Emergent reading opportunities for AAC users may be different to those given to non-AAC users. Those with physical disabilities may be unable to self-select books. Communication difficulties may mean choices are presented to them less frequently, and books are instead selected by the adults. Non-AAC users are likely to choose a small selection of books, over and over, whereas AAC users are likely to be presented with a wider range of books chosen for them. Adults are also more likely to control and dominate the conversation. The repetition of familiar books has been shown to be advantageous for literacy development (Light and McNaughton, 2020).

To develop literacy skills, AAC users need:

- Independent access to reading materials.
- Frequent opportunities for emergent writing experiences.
- Regular, planned literacy teaching which focuses on both whole word reading and decoding.
- Access to books with repetitive lines.
- Access to high frequency words via a word wall or word bank.
- Motivating supports to encourage writing, such as photographs of life events which reduce the cognitive load of having to think and plan their writing.
- Opportunities to engage in shared writing, where the adult provides scaffolding around new skills.

(Light and McNaughton, 2020)

To be able to participate in literacy learning, AAC users are likely to need adaptations to traditional approaches and resources, as they may not be able to demonstrate skills via the use of speech or handwriting. Readers who are able to use speech can demonstrate their abilities by reading words aloud. For people who are non-speaking, they can use the following strategies:

- The person reads the word and then instead of saying the word, signs it, selects a picture or symbol.

- The person is shown a picture, then selects the corresponding written word from a range of choices.
- The person hears a word, then selects the correct written form from a selection.

(Light and McNaughton, 2020; Mandak, Light and Boyle, 2018)

Phonics learning is likely to be a challenge. As the AAC user is unlikely to be able to sound out words, they will need to do this in their head (Light and McNaughton (2020), use the term *sub-vocally*). Adults can support this by sounding out the words for them, emphasising each sound.

Alternative pencils can be used to support writing practice. This could take the form of a physical pencil, which might need to be bigger to allow the person to grip, or it might be using alternative writing tools such as magnetic letters, letter cards, alphabet charts or keyboards (physical or onscreen).

Communication aids using graphic symbols will usually pair the symbol with written text, above or below. Additionally, on powered communication aids either the written text in isolation appears in the message window along the top of the screen as symbols are selected, or the symbol and text combined will appear. The assumption is often made that this supports whole word reading, however, Caron, Light and McNaughton (2020) explain how this "may pose an unintentional challenge to acquisition of sight words and, overall, to more positive literacy outcomes for individuals who require the use of AAC to communicate" (p. 117). They propose a more dynamic approach, where first the graphic symbol is selected, followed by the written text appearing separately, via animation (dynamically), and pausing on screen for three seconds. The suggestion is that a selection of words would be selected to use this feature, not every word in the AAC user's vocabulary. Producing the written text dynamically in this way may support developing links between the graphic symbol, spoken word and written word (Caron, Light and McNaughton, 2020). While their study suggested that communication aid software should adopt this feature, it is not yet widely used.

For detailed guidance around literacy learning for AAC users, see Erickson & Koppenhaver (2020) and Jane Farrall's website www.janefarrall.com/

Tips for supporting emergent readers and writers who use AAC (page 1 of 2)

People at the emergent stage of literacy will be working towards:

- Being able to identify most of the letters of the alphabet, most of the time.
- Engaging with shared reading.
- Understanding that print has meaning.

If the person can't use a pencil to practice writing, there are some alternatives listed below:

- Mark making in sand or with paint.
- Magnetic letters or printed letters on cards that they can move around.
- Chunky pencils or pens.
- A paper alphabet chart they can choose letters from. They might select using finger pointing, eye pointing, or partner-assisted scanning.
- A computer or tablet with an onscreen keyboard. They might use their hands, a switch, an adapted mouse, a joystick or an eye tracker to select the letters.
- A computer or tablet with an external keyboard. There are lots of different styles of keyboards available is standard keyboards are tricky to use.

Shared reading

Plan opportunities to share books together, daily if possible. The books might only have pictures, or some simple text. Point out the words as you read. Allow the person to choose the book themselves. Books with repetitive lines and rhyming words are great!

Shared writing

Provide materials to allow the person to practice mark making and using letters (see the list above). Use motivating experiences as a subject for their writing. It could be labelling photos of their family, or writing the names of favourite TV characters. You could write a sentence and leave a blank word for them to complete. Spelling and letter formation don't matter, it's about having fun!

Tips for supporting emergent readers and writers who use AAC (page 2 of 2)

Alphabet and phonological awareness

It's helpful to focus on one letter each day to develop the link between the sound and the letter. Look for words around you that start with that sound, you could make a book together! If the person can't say the sounds themselves, you say it for them and encourage them: "Say it in your head". Counting out syllables and finding rhyming words are also useful activities.

Independent writing with access to the full alphabet

Make sure the person is given a way they can use letters throughout the day. If they can't use a pencil, use one or more of the alternatives listed above. Encourage them to practice writing words, but don't worry about the spelling at this stage.

Self-directed reading

Allow the person to choose what they'd like to read. It doesn't have to just be books, it could be food labels, comics, posters or websites. It might be above their current level and that's ok, you can read with them. Online videos and TV programmes with captions that highlight the words as they are spoken are great!

Ideas inspired by the book Comprehensive Literacy for All: Teaching Students with Significant Disabilities to Read and Write *by Karen Erickson and David Koppenhaver, 2020, Brookes Publishing.*

Tips for supporting literacy for people who use AAC (page 1 of 2)

People at this stage of literacy development will already be able to:

- Identify most of the letters of the alphabet, most of the time.
- Engage with shared reading.
- Understand that print has meaning.

If the person can't use a pencil to practice writing, there are some alternatives listed below:

- Mark making in sand or with paint.
- Magnetic letters or printed letters on cards that they can move around.
- Chunky pencils or pens.
- A paper alphabet chart they can choose letters from. They might select using finger pointing, eye pointing or partner-assisted scanning.
- A computer or tablet with an onscreen keyboard. They might use their hands, a switch, an adapted mouse, a joystick or an eye tracker to select the letters.
- A computer or tablet with an external keyboard. There are lots of different styles of keyboards available is standard keyboards are tricky to use.

Readers who are able to use speech can demonstrate their abilities by reading words aloud. For people who are non-speaking, they can use the following strategies:

- The person reads the word and then instead of saying the word, signs it, selects a picture or symbol.
- The person is shown a picture, then selects the corresponding written word from a range of choices.
- The person hears a word, then selects the correct written word from a selection.

Reading comprehension

Provide the person with something to read and give them a question to find the answer to such as "Where did they go?" or "How did she feel?"

Tips for supporting literacy for people who use AAC (page 2 of 2)

Word study

This is about learning that words can have patterns or families, for example, words ending in "ide" - ride, hide, tide, slide. Provide activities that encourage the person to find groups of words and swap letters to make new words. It is also about learning that some words don't have patterns and need to be learned "by sight". Producing a "word wall" or chart with the words they are learning is helpful.

Writing

Provide opportunities for writing practice daily. Give the person a topic to write about or a starter question such as: "What was your best day ever?" Focus on encouragement and support, without the expectation of perfect spelling or grammar. Give positive feedback about the content of their writing such as: "I can really imagine being at the seaside with you!"

Self-directed reading

Allow the person to choose what they read. This could be scheduled reading time each day, or looking for opportunities while out and about.

Ideas inspired by the book Comprehensive Literacy for All: Teaching Students with Significant Disabilities to Read and Write *by Karen Erickson and David Koppenhaver, 2020, Brookes Publishing.*

Finding opportunities to use AAC (page 1 of 3)

Augmentative and Alternative Communication (AAC) can help people to express themselves. This might be through a paper symbol book, or software with symbols on a computer that speaks (a communication aid). When we are helping someone to learn how to use AAC, it's helpful to think about situations or "opportunities" where their AAC would be helpful.

We should avoid offering any kind of reward in exchange for using AAC. This includes strategies like:

- **Sabotage:** Pretending to forget things, or intentionally doing something wrong. For example, not putting the cutlery on the table at tea time.
- **Challenges:** Making situations difficult, such as screwing a lid on tightly, or putting something out of reach.
- **Crumbs:** Offering small pieces of a reward. For example, giving one chocolate button and waiting for the person to ask for "more".

The reasons we don't do this are because:

- Using AAC can feel like a "task" that has to be done, rather than the person associating it with genuine communication. It can quickly become boring!
- It created a power relationship, where the communication partner is in charge. They choose when the AAC user gets their reward. Interactions should be equal!
- It can cause frustration, especially if the person is new to using AAC. Knowing that there is a reward "waiting" for them after they use their AAC isn't a nice feeling, especially if they're not sure where to find a word or phrase.
- It can lead to AAC being used only in certain situations. The person might see the activity as a game and learn the rules, for example, if I press this, I get that. They might not then generalise the AAC to other situations.
- It teaches the person to be compliant. They learn to accept that they must do something to please an adult (and get their reward!). This can lead to the person being passive and compliant in other situations.

Finding opportunities to use AAC (page 2 of 3)

Instead of setting up situations when AAC use is met with a reward, we need to focus on modelling the AAC. In the same way we would speak to a young child for a year or more before we expect them to start using spoken words, we need to model AAC to the person before they will use it. We might also compare it to learning another language. This is easiest when we immerse ourselves in the language (think about having French lessons for one hour per week compared to living in France for a month!).

We model through natural situations, without expectation.

There will be opportunities to model language throughout the day. Spend some time considering the following:

- What messages is the person already able to communication using other strategies?
- What things are they struggling to communicate?
- If they were using speech, what messages would they say?
- What might be really important to them to be able to communicate? (It's important to consider messages we don't always want to hear, not just happy things!)

HOW TO MODEL WITHOUT REWARDS

Instead of ...	*Try this ...*
Pretending to drop the glue on the floor without noticing to get the person to ask for "help".	Have the glue available. Model the word "glue" when the person uses it. If they can't get the lid off, model "help".
Asking the person to request food by labelling the item or by using their AAC to say "more".	Having all snack items freely available. Model the words for the items, along with words like "want" and "more".
Hiding favourite fidget toys in a bag and waiting for the person to ask for something.	Have all the items available. As the person explores the items, model language to describe them, e.g., squishy, stretchy, bouncy.

Finding opportunities to use AAC (Page 3 of 3)

Top tips for modelling!

- **Model without expectation.** There should be no pressure to use the AAC. It can be tempting to ask them to use their AAC, but this can make AAC seem like a task or something they need to do to please you. It might take a while before they use it.
- **Keep it natural.** We all learn communication through experiencing it in everyday situations. Avoid offering rewards for using AAC, the interaction with you should be all the motivation the person needs!
- **Choose powerful language.** Think about what they would say if they were using speech. This might be words relating to their favourite things (e.g., names of books or TV characters) or it might be phrases to get their message across quickly (e.g., "go away!" or "too noisy!").
- **Accept all ways of communicating.** If a person has managed to get their message across using other strategies, we can still model that message on their AAC, but don't ask them to repeat themselves using the AAC. This can be really frustrating!
- **Model key words.** We might simplify our spoken language to a level the person can understand and then choose a few of those words to model on the AAC. For example, we might say "Lucy's gone to the shops" and then with the AAC we could model "Lucy go shop".
- **Keep the connection.** Don't put pressure on yourself to model all the time. It's better to model less and focus on the quality of the interaction. If you're putting all your effort into finding words on the AAC, they person can quickly lose interest!

What is Gestalt Language Processing Theory?

Theories suggest that some people might learn language by first understanding and using single words, then combining them to make phrases. Next, they develop the grammar and connect words to make longer messages. This is a bit like starting with single bricks (words) and building a wall (sentences). This is known as ***analytical language processing***.

Some people might learn language in "chunks". They hear a sentence and give it meaning as a whole chunk, without understanding the meaning of each word. For example, they might associate "round and round we go!" with the idea of "fun" because they love it when mum spins them on a roundabout and says "round and round we go!". They might they say "round and round we go!" whenever they are experiencing something fun. They aren't talking about the roundabout, but telling you they're enjoying themselves. This is known as ***gestalt language processing.***

We think it's common for people to use a bit of both language learning styles. They might tend to use more of one style than the other, but it's not a case of being a gestalt language learner or an analytical language learner.

If someone is non-speaking (not using any speech), or minimally speaking (only using a bit of speech) it can be hard to know if they are learning language through chunks. Here are some signs they might be:

- They love people to say certain phrases over and over again.
- They watch or listen to favourite films, programmes or YouTube videos.
- They might hum or vocalise in a tuneful "sing-song" way.

Augmentative and Alternative Communication (AAC) can help people to express themselves. This might be through a paper symbol book, or software with symbols on a computer that speaks (a communication aid).

Gestalt Language Processors and AAC

Augmentative and Alternative Communication (AAC) can help people to express themselves. This might be through a paper symbol book, or software with symbols on a computer that speaks (a communication aid).

This is how gestalt language processors might be best supported to learn to use AAC:

- **Start with powerful language.** Pick some chunks of language (phrases) that you think are really exciting for them. Consider phrases from favourite TV shows or songs and add these to their AAC.
- **Break down the chunks.** If the person starts to use the AAC with the phrases we've given them, we can try breaking down the bigger chunks into smaller ones. If one of their chunks is "round and round we go", we can break it down into "round and round" and "we go", then model these in different situations.
- **Build the chunks back up.** We can mix smaller chunks together to make new phrases. For example; "We go" + "splishy splashy".

- **Keep the gestalts!** Even if someone has started to break down their bigger chunks and join chunks together, they might still rely on their original chunks at any point in their life.
- **Add some single words:** Many symbol AAC systems use what is known as "core" and "fringe" words. Core words are words that people tend to use a lot (like "want", "go" and "me"). Fringe words are words to do with topics (like food, tv programmes and people). We can model these alongside the chunks of language.

Modelling AAC for Gestalt Language Processors

Augmentative and Alternative Communication (AAC) can help people to express themselves. This might be through a paper symbol book, or software with symbols on a computer that speaks (a communication aid). If we think someone is learning language through gestalt language processing, we can help by doing the following:

- **Choose a voice.** If it's a communication aid that speaks, see if they respond better to the voice from the communication aid (the synthetic voice), or to a recording of your own voice (most communication aids will let you record your voice onto the symbols).
- **Model the phrase.** Either pointing to the symbol and saying the phrase if it's paper AAC, or by pressing the button on the communication aid.
- **Say it once.** If you are using a communication aid that speaks (either with a synthesised or recorded voice), avoid saying the phrase as well as pressing the communication aid. Hearing it from two places can be too much!
- **Model without expectation.** There should be no pressure to use the AAC. It can be tempting to ask them to use their AAC, but this can make AAC seem like a task or something they need to do to make others happy. Communication should be natural, not forced!
- **Keep it natural.** We all learn communication through experiencing it in everyday situations. Avoid offering rewards for using AAC, the interaction with you should be all the motivation the person needs!
- **Model alternatives.** Some chunks are really hard to break down or mix together! In these cases, we model other phrases that would fit the situation. For example, if someone says "to infinity and beyond!" to show excitement, we could model "this is fun!".
- **Model as if they were saying it.** Avoid asking questions or modelling phrases with 'you' in them. For example, model "I am jumping" instead of "you like jumping!".

World

For many years, powered communication aids were both viewed and used as dedicated communication devices, meaning they had one purpose and nothing further was either possible or considered. However, over recent decades, the use of powered communication aids beyond face-to-face interactions has developed rapidly. Just as non-AAC users are now fully immersed in an online world, AAC users are embracing the benefits of digital technologies.

The use of communication aids beyond face-to-face communication is sometimes seen as a helpful way to practice new access methods, because of the lower risk associated if the user selects a target unintentionally. Choosing the wrong TV channel might be less upsetting than communicating an unintended message. Another reason for practicing access methods beyond communication is the motivational factor. While a new AAC vocabulary package might seem overwhelming to some, the opportunity to control the family television is often highly rewarding!

Computer access

Using a powered communication aid for things other than in-person communication is often referred to as "computer access". Broadly speaking, this refers to activities beyond voice output communication. This might previously have meant closing the communication software and accessing the operating system, but nowadays many AAC software have the ability to access other applications from within the application itself.

Computer control

The term "computer control" is often used to describe the process of the user controlling applications within the operating system, such as opening files on the hard drive, viewing documents, word processing and sending email. Usually, the software will present a control panel which allows the user to use functions such as single or double click, right or left click, scroll and tab. This occurs over the computer desktop.

Accessible apps

Some AAC software might use to "accessible apps". These are pages constructed within the communication software that allow the user control of an external app, such as Netflix or Instagram. These won't look exactly like the app displayed on a computer, tablet or smartphone, but will present it in a way that is easier for AAC users to control. Apps are accessed from within the communication pages. A common challenge is when the app developers make changes to the app, which is not immediately noticed by the AAC software developer and the accessible app stops working until an update is created and released.

Phone calls and texting

Most AAC software will allow for text messaging and phone calls. The person's mobile phone is connected via Bluetooth, and text messages are viewed and composed via pages within the communication software. Telephone calls can also be made via the communication software, playing the conversation from the communication aid speakers rather than the handset.

The internet and social media

It is now typical for powered communication aids to have access to the internet, which brings with it the opportunity to engage with social media. AAC users have reported that putting a message on social media makes it easy to communicate to lots of people at once, rather than having to repeat the message over and over in a face-to-face interaction (Caron and Light, 2016).

AAC users report that communicating through social media can be easier than in-person interactions. One reason for this is the reduction in time-pressure. Social media interactions allow for asynchronous communication, where messages might be exchanged with long gaps in between each turn, reducing the demand to formulate a message "in the moment".

Messages conveyed online don't always reply on text. It's now common for social media users to convey concepts through images, such as photographs, GIFs and memes (Light and McNaughton, 2014).

The multimodal nature of online interactions, along with an asynchronous communication style, means that AAC users report that they are better able to portray their true identity and feel "typical". Indeed, they may not reveal the fact they an AAC user at all should they decide not to. Their communication partner may not be aware of their communication difficulties or differences, in stark contrast to face-to-face interactions. AAC users have reported perceiving that other people are more willing to engage with them online than in person (Caron and Light, 2016). Use of social media can result in people feeling they can portray a more accurate picture of their true self (Hynan, Murray and Goldbart, 2014). Many other advantages of social media use have been written about, including increased independence, being able to seek help and support and gaining employment (Caron and Light, 2016; Hynan, Murray and Goldbart, 2014; Light and McNaughton, 2014).

AAC users may also face barriers to successful social media use. This might first occur at the point of obtaining a communication aid, as some services may block or restrict internet use. If internet access is allowed, practitioners supporting the individual might not possess the skills to support social media use, or might not see it as part of their role.

Access needs may be an additional barrier to successful use of social media, either through physical access to the technology, or through limitations of software.

If users do not have good literacy skills, they are likely to need a high level of support from friends, family or practitioners to engage with social media platforms. Aside from social media, the internet offers communication aid users with the potential for increased independence through things like internet banking, online shopping and booking systems.

Gaming

For many years, access to mainstream gaming platforms such as Microsoft Xbox and Sony PlayStation® was rarely considered for AAC users with complex access needs. However, in recent years this is has become increasingly possible. Games developers are building an increasing number of accessibility options into their games. There are an ever-increasing range of alternative controllers, with even Microsoft and Sony themselves developing alternative console controllers.

The solutions are varied and can be complex. It would not be appropriate to highlight any particular solutions here as the pace of change is swift, however the details of the UK-based charity Special Effect who specialise in alternative access methods for gaming are given here, along with their blog which covers video game accessibility resources:

Special Effect Charity: www.specialeffect.org.uk/

Game Access Blog: https://gameaccess.info/

Environmental control

Environmental control, often abbreviated to "EC", refers to the use of assistive technology to control items within the person's environment. This can include:

- Remote plug sockets, allowing control of anything with an "on/off" function, such as a fan, blender, bubble tube or lamp
- Automatic door, blind and curtain openers
- Door intercoms
- Mains powered lighting
- Landline telephones
- Heating
- Televisions, DVD players, radios and stereos
- Control of home automation systems
- Telecare services (personal alarms).

Environmental control technology works in one of the following ways:

- Infrared (IR), which requires direct line of sight to work (like a TV remote control).
- Radio frequency (RF), which can work through walls and does not require line of sight.

Sometimes, adaptations might need to be made to the person's home, usually when mains lighting or door, curtain and blind openers are required. The person may need to pay for these adaptations themselves.

Due to technological advances and the increasing use of virtual assistants in the home (e.g., Amazon Echo, Apple's Siri and Google Assistant), functions which previously might have required a specialist environmental control device or communication aid are now achievable through mainstream technology.

Points to consider

When offering environmental control, computer access and gaming, there are some key points to consider:

- If someone is given a long list of everything that is possible, they may feel obliged to accept the options, or be excited by the seemingly endless possibilities. In reality, they might only use one or two key functions (that's not to say that people don't use the whole range of functions available!). It is often a good idea to pick one or two important functions for the person, start with those and then add more later if desired.

- When choosing functions to trial, it's important to consider the person's previous awareness and use of these technologies. Have they ever used internet banking before? Are they already familiar with YouTube? If not, is there sufficient support around them to help learn new skills? Some charities may support with this.
- Usernames, passwords and accounts can often be a barrier to setting these systems up. If you are going to visit a person to help with these things, ask them to have their existing email address, user names and passwords to hand. If they are alone, they will likely need to disclose these personal details to you.
- Safeguarding should be a consideration, especially when setting up internet access for someone. Consideration should be given as to whether they are able to use and manage online payments, whether internet browsing should be limited or supervised, and who they might be able to interact with while online. For some people, the camera and/or webcam may need to be disabled.

Summary

In this chapter we have considered how we support AAC users to learn to use their AAC. This includes practicing the access method such as switch scanning or eye pointing. There are frameworks that can help to guide this process. It's important to involve the AAC user and their family in selecting the words and phrases that are added to their AAC. This might involve having some challenging conversations. The balance of words and phrases might look very different depending on whether the person uses a predominantly analytical or gestalt style of learning language.

We need to provide opportunities to practice using words, without relying on approaches which teach compliance, using only natural prompts. We must also provide access to literacy, as this opens up many opportunities for the AAC user.

Finally, if the person is using powered AAC, we should think beyond face-to-face communication and provide opportunities to use social media, texting and gaming. There might also be the option to control appliances witing their environment, such as the television or lighting.

References

Adams, M. J. (1994). Beginning to read: Thinking and learning about print.

Ahern, K. (2016, March 24). Rethinking the AAC prompting hierarchy in severe apraxia. *Teaching Learners with Multiple Special Needs*. http://teachinglearnerswithmultipleneeds.blogspot.com/2016/03/rethinking-aac-prompting-hierarchy-in.html.

Ahern, K. (2023, November 10). Revisiting the adapted AAC prompt hierarchy – Seven years later. *AAC Voices BEE HEARD!!* www.aacvoices.org/blog/aac-prompt-hierarchy.

Ahlgrim-Delzell, L., Browder, D. M., Wood, L., Stanger, C., Preston, A. I. and Kemp-Inman, A. (2016). Systematic instruction of phonics skills using an iPad for students with developmental disabilities who are AAC users. *The Journal of Special Education*, 50(2), 86–97. https://doi.org/10.1177/0022466915622140.

Barker, M. R., Saunders, K. J. and Brady, N. C. (2012). Reading instruction for children who use AAC: Considerations in the pursuit of generalizable results. *Augmentative and Alternative Communication*, 28(3), 160–170. https://doi.org/10.3109/07434618.2012.704523.

Battye, A. (2023). *Navigating AAC: 50 Essential Strategies and Resources for Using Augmentative and Alternative Communication*. Routledge.

Bean, Ian. (2011). *Switch Progression Learning Journeys Road Map* [Computer software]. www.ianbean.co.uk/Downloads/SPRM.pdf.

Beukelman, D. and Mirenda, P. (2005). *Augmentative & Alternative Communication*. Paul H Brooks Publishing.

Biederman, G. B., Fairhall, J. L., Raven, K. A. and Davey, V. A. (1998). Verbal Prompting, hand-over-hand instruction, and passive observation in teaching children with developmental disabilities. *Exceptional Children*, 64(4), 503–511. https://doi.org/10.1177/001440299806400406.

Blanc, M., Blackwell, A. and Elias, P. (2023). Using the natural language acquisition protocol to support gestalt language development. *Perspectives of the ASHA Special Interest Groups*, 1–8. https://doi.org/10.1044/2023_PERSP-23-00098.

Burkhart, L. (2018). Stepping stones to switch access. *Perspectives of the ASHA Special Interest Groups*, 3, 33–44. https://lindaburkhart.com/wp-content/uploads/2018/06/ASHA_Persepctives_Switches_Burkhart.pdf.

Caron, J. and Light, J. (2016). Social media has opened a world of "Open communication": Experiences of adults with cerebral palsy who use Augmentative and Alternative Communication and social media. *Augmentative and Alternative Communication*, 32(1), 25–40. https://doi.org/10.3109/07434618.2015.1052887.

Caron, J., Light, J. and McNaughton, D. (2020). Effects of an AAC app with transition to literacy features on single-word reading of individuals with complex communication needs. *Research and Practice for Persons with Severe Disabilities*, 45(2), 115–131. https://doi.org/10.1177/1540796920911152.

Chandler, R. J., Russell, A. and Maras, K. L. (2019). Compliance in autism: Self-report in action. *Autism*, 23(4), 1005–1017. https://doi.org/10.1177/1362361318795479.

Clarke, M. T., Sargent, J., Cooper, R., Aberbach, G., McLaughlin, L., Panesar, G., Woghiren, A., Griffiths, T., Price, K., Rose, C. and Swettenham, J. (2022). Development and testing of the eye-pointing classification scale for children with cerebral palsy. *Disability and Rehabilitation*, 44(8), 1451–1456. https://doi.org/10.1080/09638288.2020.1800834.

Clendon, S. and Anderson, K. (2016). Syntax and morphology in aided language development. In M. M. Smith and J. Murray (eds) *The Silent Partner? Language, Interaction and Aided Communication* (pp. 119–140). J & R Press Ltd.

Da Fonte, M. A. and Boesch, M. C. (2018). *Effective Augmentative and Alternative Communication Practices: A Handbook for School-based Practitioners*. Routledge.

Erickson, K. and Koppenhaver, D. (2020). *Comprehensive Literacy for All: Teaching Students with Significant Disabilities to Read and Write*. Brookes Publishing.

Griffiths, T., Clarke, M. T. and Swettenham, J. (2023). The ability of typically developing 2–3-year-olds to infer the control mechanism for eye-gaze technology and the impact of causal language instruction. *Disability and Rehabilitation: Assistive Technology*, 19(7), 1–8. https://doi.org/10.1080/17483107.2023.2293874.

Hynan, A., Murray, J. and Goldbart, J. (2014). "Happy and excited": Perceptions of using digital technology and social media by young people who use augmentative and alternative communication. *Child Language Teaching and Therapy*, 30(2), 175–186. https://doi.org/10.1177/0265659013519258.

Judge, S. and Colven, D. (2006). Switch access to technology – A comprehensive guide. Computer Science.

Karlsson, P., Griffiths, T., Clarke, M. T., Monbaliu, E., Himmelmann, K., Bekteshi, S., Allsop, A., Pereksles, R., Galea, C. and Wallen, M. (2021). Stakeholder consensus for decision making in eye-gaze control technology for children, adolescents and adults with cerebral palsy service provision: Findings from a Delphi study. *BMC Neurology*, 21(1), 63. https://doi.org/10.1186/s12883-021-02077-z.

Koppenhaver, D. (2000). Literacy in AAC: What should be written on the envelope we push? *Augmentative and Alternative Communication*, 16(4), 270–279. https://doi.org/10.1080/07434610012331279124.

Langley, R. (2023, February 19). Revisiting the Prompt Hierarchy for AAC. Canva.Com. www.canva.com/design/DAFbT9-6ExE/bdRp7SVEZ4psml7c2-2i4Q/view?utm_content=DAFbT9-6ExE&utm_campaign=designshare&utm_medium=link&utm_source=publishsharelink#2.

Light, J. and McNaughton, D. (2014). Communicative competence for Individuals who require Augmentative and Alternative Communication: A new definition for a new era of communication? *Augmentative and Alternative Communication*, 30(1), 1–18. https://doi.org/10.3109/07434618.2014.885080.

Light, J. C. and McNaughton, D. B. (2020). Literacy intervention for individuals with complex communication needs. In D. R. Beukelman and P. Mirenda, *Augmentative & Alternative Communication: Supporting Children and Adults with Complex Communication Needs* (pp. 427–480). Brookes Publishing.

Mandak, K., Light, J. and Boyle, S. (2018). The effects of literacy interventions on single-word reading for individuals who use aided AAC: A systematic review. *Augmentative and Alternative Communication*, 34(3), 206–218. https://doi.org/10.1080/07434618.2018.1470668.

McCarthy, J., McCarthy, J., Light, J., Drager, K., McNaughton, D., Grodzicki, L., Jones, J., Panek, E. and Parkin, E. (2006). Re-designing scanning to reduce learning demands: The performance of typically developing 2-year-olds. *Augmentative and Alternative Communication*, 22(4), 269–283. https://doi.org/10.1080/00498250600718621.

Money, D. (1997). A comparison of three approaches to delivering a speech and language therapy service to people with learning disabilities. *International Journal of Language & Communication Disorders*, 32(4), 449–466. https://doi.org/10.3109/13682829709082259.

Moorcroft, A., Scarinci, N. and Meyer, C. (2021). "I've had a love-hate, I mean mostly hate relationship with these PODD books": Parent perceptions of how they and their child contributed to AAC rejection and abandonment. *Disability and Rehabilitation: Assistive Technology*, 16(1), 72–82. https://doi.org/10.1080/17483107.2019.1632944.

O'Neill, T., Light, J. and Pope, L. (2018). Effects of interventions that include aided Augmentative and Alternative Communication input on the communication of individuals with complex communication needs: A meta-analysis. *Journal of Speech, Language, and Hearing Research*, 61(7), 1743–1765. https://doi.org/10.1044/2018_JSLHR-L-17-0132.

Robinson, H. (2023) The Positive AAC Framework [Poster presentation], Communication Matters Conference, 12 September, 2023.

Sturm, J. M., Erickson, K. and Yoder, D. E. (2002). Enhancing literacy development through AAC technologies. *Assistive Technology*, 14(1), 71–80. https://doi.org/10.1080/10400435.2002.10132056.

7

PLANNING

Helen Robinson

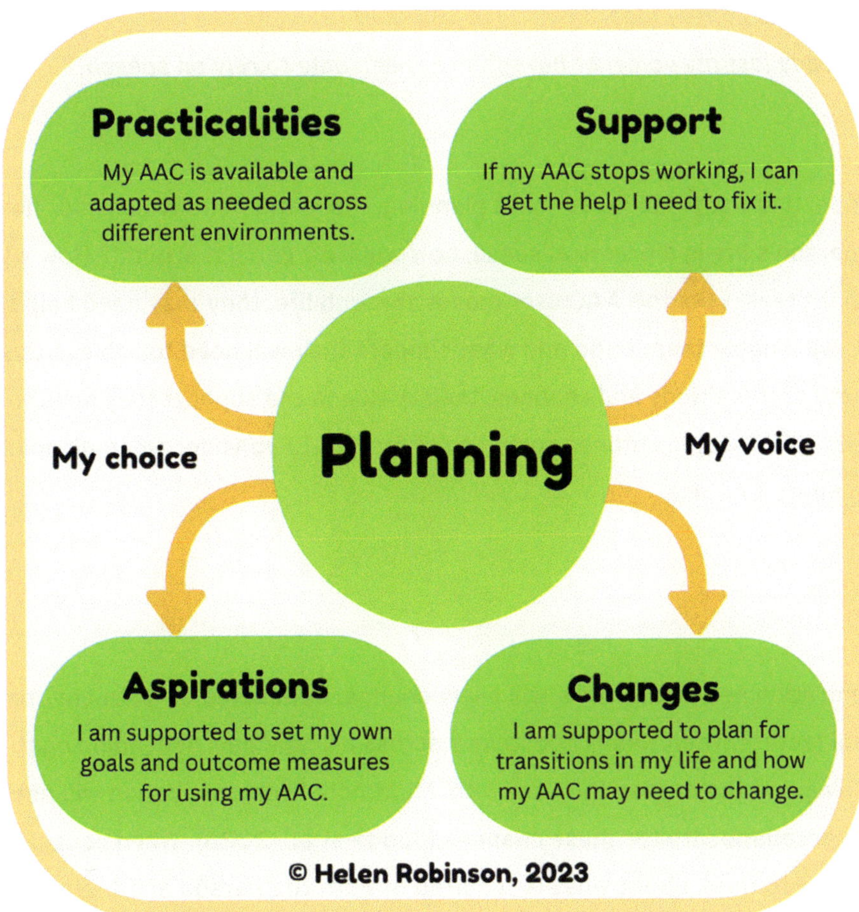

Figure 7.1 The planning strand from The Positive AAC Framework
Source: Robinson (2023).

DOI: 10.4324/9781003412311-9

Using AAC and supporting people to do so takes planning. Plans will need to consider how AAC will fit into a person's life in a practical sense; how will they carry it around? How will they get help when it breaks? As the AAC user moves through life, they may need help to consider what AAC will enable them to do and what support they will need to achieve this. As they face a variety of transitions and changes, their AAC and the support they need will likely need to adapt. This chapter outlines some of the factors to consider when planning to introduce and support AAC use.

Practicalities

A person's communication needs and skills will likely change, depending on both environmental and personal factors. Their needs might vary across a single day, depending on the activity they are doing and the person they are with. Multimodal communication will need to be considered to accommodate for these changes (Judge et al., 2023). When considering AAC, it's important to think about what is required of both the person and their environment in order to use it successfully. Some factors are summarised in Table 7.1.

Table 7.1 Practical considerations for AAC use

Factors which might impact AAC use	*Practical considerations*	*Questions to ask*
Battery life	Batteries on powered communication aids can last up to ten hours, but might run out quicker with constant use. Additional battery packs or power banks can be purchased for most powered AAC. Magnetic charging leads can be useful for people who need to charge their communication aid independently.	Is there access to a charging point? Is there someone available to charge the communication aid? Do they know how to charge it? Does the person need to be able to connect a charger themselves?
Wheelchairs, seating and postural equipment	The weight and position of a communication aid may be significant when mounting to some equipment. There is a risk if the equipment tipping over or the communication aid hitting things like doorframes if mounted outside the footprint of the wheelchair. Some equipment will not have a suitable point to fix a mount to.	Is there a point to fix the mount? Can the equipment be used safely while the communication aid is mounted? Does the person need to put their communication aid on and off the mount independently?
Sunlight	If using AAC outside, sunlight can impact some access methods. Some eye trackers will not be effective outside, although many newer trackers are able to compensate for bright light. Screen glare, or glare from laminated paper may be an issue. Matt laminate can be used to minimise this.	Will the person be outside often and if so, will their choice of AAC need to change?
Rain and water	Environments which expose the communication aid to water can be problematic, either in terms of getting electrical equipment wet, or unlaminated paper.	Will the AAC be used outside often? What AAC will they use when in the bathroom?
Space	If a person is in a small space, which might be their home, education or work setting, sometimes floor mounts can be problematic. Mounts with different bases, such as flat plates, can be helpful to slide under furniture. If someone isn't available to move the mount between rooms, the person may need to be provided with several mounts (e.g., one in the bedroom and one in the kitchen).	If a floor mount is required, will it fit in the room? How is the room used? Will the communication aid need to be moved around the room, or between rooms? Is there someone to move the mount?
Other people	Busy classrooms can sometimes present hazards, both to the AAC user and those around them.	Is anyone likely to pull or swing on the mount or the AAC (if mounted)? Is anyone likely to take the AAC and throw it?
Personal safety	AAC users who travel independently may either be at risk of their communication aid being stolen, or feel vulnerable if their communication aid is visible.	Does the communication aid need to be covered or hidden in a bag at any time?

(*Continued*)

Table 7.1 Continued

Factors which might impact AAC use	*Practical considerations*	*Questions to ask*
Carrying the AAC	If the person needs to hold and carry their AAC themselves, they may need to fit it in a bag or a pocket or use a carry strap.	Does the person need to carry the communication aid independently?
Support available	Confidence and skill in supporting different AAC methods will vary across setting and consequently, if might not be possible for the person to use either a particular mode of AAC, or access method, in particular settings.	What level of support is available in each setting? Might different modes of AAC need to be used in different places?
Fatigue	A person might be sleepy in the morning, or fatigue as the day goes on. This can impact the mode of AAC they are able to use.	Does the type of AAC, or the access method need to change throughout the day?
Glasses	A person might switch between wearing glasses and not. This might affect some access methods, such as eye trackers.	Does the person wear glasses and will this impact their AAC use?
Experiencing periods of mutism or being semi speaking	Autistic AAC users may experience periods of mutism. This can not only impact their use of speech, but might also affect their ability to spell, hold AAC, look at a screen, or compose messages.	Does the person need access to the alphabet, symbols or pre-stored phrases? Does the person need to use alternative access methods at times (such partner assisted scanning)?

The handout *Communication aid set-up guide* can be used to inform those supporting the person in how to set up their communication aid and access method. There are headings relating only to powered communication aids, but these can be omitted if the AAC is paper based. The handout *How to help me communicate* can be useful to provide alongside the set-up guide, or in place of it if powered AAC isn't being used.

Communication aid set-up guide

Name:	
Model of communication aid:	
Name of the software on my communication aid:	
Name of the vocabulary pages on my communication aid:	

<table>
<tr><td>The name I use to refer to my communication aid:</td><td></td></tr>
<tr><td colspan="2">Insert photograph of the communication aid. It is a good idea to label the power button, volume button and charging port</td></tr>
<tr><td>How I control my communication aid:</td><td>insert description of access method, including any settings such as scan pattern and speech for switches or dwell time for eye trackers</td></tr>
<tr><td colspan="2">insert photograph of the person using their communication aid to show the access method and positioning</td></tr>
<tr><td>How to position my communication aid:</td><td></td></tr>
</table>

Details of mounting equipment for my communication aid:	*Insert details of how to set up the mount, and any safety information* *insert link to mounting manual, user guide and/or website*
Insert photographs of any mounts	
How to charge my communication aid:	
Name of the person who will charge my communication aid:	
How to start up and shut down my communication aid:	
How to clean my communication aid:	

Name of the company/person to call if my communication aid isn't working:	
Contact details for the company/person:	

Support

Planning the support that a person needs when introducing AAC can be challenging. The AAC user and the people around them might not be able to identify what support they will need before trialling AAC. In their longitudinal study of AAC users receiving communication aids, Broomfield et al. noted that "the concept of 'support' may not always be practical but may take the shape of increasing communicative opportunity, nurturing a nourishing environment, or even prompting individual motivation" (2023, p. 21).

If a person is using a powered communication aid, it's important that they and those supporting them know how to seek help if it stops working. The *Communication aid support plan* can be used to inform everyone of what to do when things go wrong.

A key factor is agreeing who is responsible for making a backup of the software, how often and how this will be stored. It's worth giving consideration to what would happen if this person were not available for any reason, and how the backup could be accessed. Communication aid software usually has a variety of ways in which it can be backed up. Settings may have policies regarding which methods can be used and which are not permitted. AAC companies will usually provide written or video instructions explaining how to make a backup.

Another consideration is what AAC method will be used if powered AAC isn't available. If powered AAC is primarily used, it can be helpful to have a paper-based AAC system available alongside this, along with other well-practices strategies.

Helping people to support AAC users is further explored in Chapter 8.

Communication aid support plan

Name	
Model of my communication aid	
Name of the software on my communication aid	
Name of the vocabulary pages on my communication aid	
Name of the company that supports my communication aid	
Contact details for the company that supports my communication aid	
Instructions for making a backup of my communication aid software and/or vocabulary pages	
Name of person/people responsible for making and storing a backup of my communication aid software and/or vocabulary pages	
Details of what to use if my communication aid isn't working	
Name of the voice on my communication aid	
Any adjustments that have been made to the voice on my communication aid (pitch, speed)	
Username	
Password	

How to help me communicate

Name	
The ways I communicate	
The way I tell you yes	
The way I tell you no	
Signs that I am happy	
Signs that I am not happy	
Things you can do to help me understand	
Things you can do to help me communicate (e.g., give me options, use objects)	
Information about how I use my person-based communication (e.g., facial expression, eye pointing, body movements, gesture, signing, speech, sounds)	
Information about how I use paper-based communication (e.g., printed symbols, an alphabet chart, a communication book)	
Information about how I use a powered communication aid (e.g., a tablet, a computer, mobile phone)	
Please do ...	
Please do not ...	

Aspirations

Understanding the aspirations of each individual can have a significant impact on their use of AAC, perhaps even preventing it from being abandoned. **Patient reported outcome measures (PROMs)** can be used to gain the views of people regarding their quality of life and impact of any interventions. Broomfield et al. (2019) found that despite this, the views of AAC users are rarely sought.

There may be barriers within the population of AAC users which make completing PROMs challenging, relating to their communication, physical and cognitive needs and, as such, creative means of gathering their views (such as visual supports) may need to be utilised. Often, outcome measures will be completed by someone else on behalf of the AAC user. While not a PROM, Talking Mats can be a useful tool to enable the opinions of AAC users to be gained (Broomfield et al., 2019).

It is common for the use of AAC in itself is seen as a successful outcome, instead of viewing AAC as a facilitator to achieving broader goals. Historically, goals were set and measured around linguistic competence. Over time, the focus has shifted first towards functional communication skills (effective communication) and then towards considering AAC in terms of participation (allowing the individual to engage with activities at home, school, work, or in the community) (Light and McNaughton, 2012).

The concept of communicative competence has long underpinned goal setting within AAC. Communicative competence essentially is a measure of how effective a person's communication is. Various interpretations and representations of communicative competence have been presented over the years, evolving from the 1980s onwards. Earlier models very much aimed for typical communication based on the communication skills on non-AAC users. Teachman and Gibson (2013) present an overview of the evolution of communicative competence over the past four decades, highlighting seven key conceptualisations. Perhaps the most well-known of these definitions is Light's model of communicative competency using the components of linguistic competency, operational competency, social competency and strategic competency (Light, 1989; Light, Beukelman and Reichle, 2003; Light and McNaughton, 2014). Light (1989) outlined that communicative competence is context dependent, influenced by the characteristics of the person, environmental factors and the characteristics of the communication partner.

Light's model of communicative competence has seen several evolutions over the past 30 years. Expanding on the initial model, the 2003 version included the addition of psychosocial factors, as follows: motivation, attitude, confidence and resilience, environmental supports and barriers, policy and practice barriers and supports, attitude barriers and supports, and knowledge and skill barriers and supports (Light, Beukelman and Reichle, 2003). The 2014 iteration recognised developments in communication aid technology, changes in the population that uses AAC, changes in the way the world communicates (moving beyond just face to face interactions, taking account of the growing use of social media and mobile technologies) and increased demands on participation for AAC users. Despite highlighting the changes that had occurred since the original 1989 model, Light and McNaughton concluded that the fundamental concepts were still applicable, stating:

> AAC interventions must address the development of adequate, functional communication skills to support individuals with complex communication needs in developing, rebuilding, or sustaining communicative competence to express needs and wants, develop social closeness, exchange information, and participate in social etiquette routines as required.
>
> *(Light and McNaughton, 2014, p. 23)*

Light's model, and others before and after it, have been praised for presenting aided communication as a difference rather than a deficit and moving away from goals of "normal" communication, however, there has also been criticism that many of these models see communicative competence being achieved (or not) by the AAC user themselves, supported by those around them, rather than competence being the collective achievement or a communication partnership or group. Teachman and Gibson argue that communicative competence is "a shared, socially incorporated and performed communication construct" (2014, p. 2) and warn of relying too heavily on models of communicative competence which are still ultimately based on perpetuated ideals of fixing and curing, stating: "for many individuals who use AAC, 'normal' standards of communication are not attainable or feasible, whereas being listened to and acknowledged as a person who is communicating differently can and should be a goal" (Teachman and Gibson, 2014, p. 10).

Over recent years, goal setting has shifted focus towards a participation model, looking at how AAC users can be better included within society, facilitated by adaptations that support communication access to everyday activities.

People's expectations of what AAC can do for them and how they will use it are likely to evolve. Some people may be unclear what they want AAC to do when they are initially provided with a communication aid. As they begin to use it and understand its benefits and limitations, they will likely form a clear idea of what they want from it.

Sometimes, people will have unrealistic expectations of what a communication aid can do. This might be the user themselves or those supporting them.

The way in which a person perceives their communication aid may change over time, as they learn to use AAC and integrate it into their daily lives. What might initially be seen as a tool to deliver key messages can evolve to become a tool to develop social bonds, express identity and enable people to participate in a range of activities (Broomfield et al., 2023).

The Communication Matters Outcome Measures Project (2012) reviewed the outcome measures currently being used by AAC services. They found that frequently assessments were being used as outcome measures and it wasn't always clear what defined an outcome measure (Murphy, 2013).

Questions to ask AAC users and/or their communication partners when setting goals:

- What do you/they struggle to talk about now that you hope AAC might help with?
- What activities do you/they hope AAC might help you to take part in?

Changes

The AAC strategies that a person uses will undoubtedly change over time, either because of changes to their needs and abilities, changes within their environment or because their communication aid reaches the end of its life (Broomfield et al., 2023). Here, we consider the changes a person might encounter under the headings of developmental, health and environmental.

Environmental changes

People will inevitably encounter changes to the environments they live within throughout their life, including:

- Changing classes at school each year
- Changing schools
- Moving into work and subsequently changing jobs
- Respite care

- Moving house (and local community)
- Moving into a nursing home
- Hospital stays

Even when the setting remains stable, changes to the people around the parson can change, including:

- Relationships ending and new ones beginning.
- Family members becoming unwell and moving out of the home.
- Death of family members and friends.
- Siblings moving out of the family home.
- Paid carers changing or leaving their role.
- Teaching professionals leaving their role, or being unwell and not at work.
- Changes to nursing staff.

Broomfield et al. (2023) describe the journey of one AAC user who initially saw his communication aid as a tool to support him at work and not use it at home, but when the COVID-19 pandemic occurred and he remained at home, the use of his communication aid in that environment increased greatly. For another person, their communication aid was less well supported at home compared to school and the pandemic saw their communication aid use reduce.

Developmental changes

As children grow, there are various ways in which this can impact their AAC use. New seating and wheelchairs will mean that any communication aids mounted will need to be re-fitted to their new equipment. As they move through adolescence and into adulthood, they may wish to change the voice on their powered communication aid, to reflect their maturity. Advancing literacy skills will mean that a child using graphic symbols will need their vocabulary package reviewing.

Health changes

A person's health can impact their ability to use AAC significantly. They might lose or gain physical or sensory abilities and their AAC might need to change to support this. The obvious change is the way in which they access their communication aid, for example, loss of hand function might mean direct access is no longer possible and switch access or eye gaze needs to be explored. Changes in their vision could mean that the font size needs increasing, or they need fewer items on a page.

People may not always be aware that alternative access methods are possible; sometimes they think that the AAC they have been provided with is the only option. This can prevent people from reporting when their AAC is no longer suitable and therefore those with degenerative conditions will need regular reviews.

Voice and message banking

If the AAC user has a degenerative condition and is likely to lose their speech, they may choose to bank their voice. Voice banking is frequently promoted to people who have motor neurone disease. Voice banking involves recording one's speech which is then used to create a personalised synthetic voice. This synthetic voice can then be downloaded onto a communication aid at any point in the future. There are a number of commercial companies that support voice banking, and most do not charge for the voice until it is downloaded. Owners of Apple products can make use of the "Personal Voice" feature, which enables them to make a 15-minute recording of their voice, which will then be converted into a synthesised voice for use on Apple devices.

The process of banking one's voice involves the person recording themselves saying a set list of words and phrases provided by the voice banking company, using a computer and microphone, via the voice banking company's website. If the person is well, this process can take a little as 20 minutes, but can take up to two hours. A synthetic voice is then produced, which will sound like the person's own voice at the time of recording. For this reason, it is best to complete voice banking as soon as possible once the person is aware they are likely to lose their own voice. This can be a difficult conversation to have with the person in the early days of receiving a diagnosis, although some people report that banking their voice can feel like a positive action during difficult times.

Some people may complete voice banking and either never need to use a synthetic voice, or they may choose not to use it for a variety of reasons. Some people can find their banked synthetic voice upsetting, or may be disappointed with the quality of it.

People may also choose to complete message banking, where they record words or phrases directly into software for use on their communication aid later on (Costello, 2016). This will be a recording of their voice, as it is now, and is not used to create a synthetic voice. People might use it to record phrases such as "I love you", or other sayings or phrases which are personal to them. The messages can be recorded in to communication aid software, which will have a cost, or via a voice banking website or app which is often free of charge. The messages will then be stored and can be added to a communication aid at a later date.

Practitioners may need to support people to bank their voices and/or messages. They will need to be confident in explaining the process to the person and their family and for this reason it is a good idea for the practitioner to complete the process of voice and/or message banking themselves. People may also need support in choosing the company or software to use, setting up an account, sourcing a microphone and setting this up and actually using the software to complete the process.

Voice repair

For people whose voice has already begun to deteriorate, a growing number of companies are offering a voice repair service. The person completes voice banking, often using fewer recorded words and phrases than the typical voice banking process. The company then blends their voice with another synthetic voice they have stored which sounds similar, and a new synthetic voice which sounds close to the person's own voice will be produced.

Synthetic voice design

Synthetic voice design is becoming more frequently used. This is useful for people who are unable to bank their own voice because it has already deteriorated, or people who have development communication differences and never used speech. If the person has previously used speech, they can provide a recording to the company who will blend this with another donor voice to produce a synthetic voice. They need at least five minutes of their voice recorded, although longer samples will produce a better-quality voice.

For people without a previous recording of their own voice, they can choose two donor voices, either from their friends and family or from the company directly. These two donor voices are then blended to produce a synthetic voice which will be unique to the individual.

Summary

In this chapter we have thought about how we can prepare someone to use AAC, provide ongoing support to use it and how their AAC might need to adapt as they move through life.

Much focus is often given to the initial AAC assessment and provision. Goals might be set for beginning AAC users, without regular, ongoing review. Often, beginning AAC users and their families won't fully understand the possibilities and limitations of AAC use and may find it tricky to set goals and outline the support they need. It is tempting to set goals and make plans on behalf of the AAC user; however, good quality support will seek the opinion of the AAC user and make use of Patient Reported Outcome Measures (PROMs).

Janice Light's definition of communicative competence is well used to support goal setting and measure progress, however there is now a shift towards more participation-based models which emphasise the impact of the role of communication partners and the person's environment.

Communication aid voices - what are my options? (page 1 of 2)

Communication aids can help people who aren't able to use their own voice for effective communication. This might be in some places, with certain people, or all of the time. There are several options when choosing the voice that speaks out the messages.

Synthetic voices

Communication aids will come with a number of in-built voices to choose from. There is a wide selection to choose from, with different regional accents. These are usually included in the price of the app or software. Most will allow you to adjust the pitch and speed of the voice if you like, to make it more unique.

Voice banking

If you currently use speech that is easy for most people to understand, you can choose to "bank" your voice. This involves you having to record a set list of words and phrases, which can take from as little as 15 minutes and up to two hours. Your recordings are then used to create a synthetic voice that sounds like you. You can bank this voice for later, should you lose your speech and need to use a communication aid. Most companies don't charge a fee to bank your voice, but might charge you to download and use it. If you have an Apple iPhone or iPad, the "Personal Voice" feature will allow you to create a synthetic voice to use on Apple devices. It's worth being aware that if you need to use a communication aid in future that is made by a different company, you won't be able to use the voice created using Apple's Personal Voice.

Message banking

Some people chose to record some messages which can be saved in a piece of software and used later on a communication aid. This isn't a synthetic voice, but simply the recording of your own voice. It can be powerful to record yourself saying messages for loved ones, such as "I love you" or any common phrases you currently use.

Communication aid voices – what are my options? (page 2 of 2)

What if my own voice isn't very clear?

If you can use speech but it isn't very clear, "voice repair" might be an option to consider. This is like voice banking, but requires fewer recorded phrases. The company will blend your voice with one of the standard synthetic voices they use, to create a unique voice for you to use on a communication aid.

What if I have already lost my voice, or haven't ever been able to rely on speech?

Synthetic voice design offers the option of creating a synthetic voice using "donor" voices. If you previously used speech and have a recording of yourself which is five minutes or longer, it is possible to use this to create a synthetic voice which sounds like you.

Another option is to select two friends or family members to complete voice banking and the company can blend these voices together to create a unique voice. If you don't have anyone willing to bank their voice, the companies can use several stored voices to create you a synthetic voice.

References

Broomfield, K., Harrop, D., Judge, S., Jones, G. and Sage, K. (2019). Appraising the quality of tools used to record patient-reported outcomes in users of Augmentative and Alternative Communication (AAC): A systematic review. *Quality of Life Research*, 28(10), 2669-2683. https://doi.org/10.1007/s11136-019-02228-3.

Broomfield, K., Judge, S., Sage, K., Jones, G. L. and James, D. (2023). Using longitudinal qualitative research to explore the experience of receiving and using Augmentative and Alternative Communication. *International Journal of Language & Communication Disorders*, 1460–6984. https://doi.org/10.1111/1460-6984.12981.

Communication Matters, 2012. Outcome Measures Project. aac_outcome_measurement_sept_2012.pdf.

Costello, J. M. (2016). Message banking vs. voice banking: A very successful proactive model for people with ALS/MND. 14th Annual Allied Professionals Forum. Dublin. www.alsmndalliance.org/wp-content/uploads/2016/12/costello-message-banking-handout.pdf.

Judge, S., Moran, C. and Randall, N. (2023). How do people who use Augmentative and Alternative Communication use multimodal communication in real-life situations? A literature review. *Communication Matters Journal*, 37(1), 26–29.

Light, J. (1989). Toward a definition of communicative competence for individuals using Augmentative and Alternative Communication systems. *Augmentative and Alternative Communication*, 5(2), 137–144. https://doi.org/10.1080/07434618912331275126.

Light, J. C., Beukelman, D. R. and Reichle, J. (eds). (2003). *Communicative Competence for Individuals Who Use AAC: From Research to Effective Practice*. Paul H. Brookes.

Light, J. and McNaughton, D. (2012). The changing face of Augmentative and Alternative Communication: Past, present, and future challenges. *Augmentative and Alternative Communication*, 28(4), 197–204. https://doi.org/10.3109/07434618.2012.737024.

Light, J. and McNaughton, D. (2014). Communicative competence for individuals who require Augmentative and Alternative Communication: A new definition for a new era of communication? *Augmentative and Alternative Communication*, 30(1), 1–18. https://doi.org/10.3109/07434618.2014.885080.

Murphy, J. (2013). *A Critical Appraisal of Existing Methods of Measuring Outcomes in Relation to Augmentative and Alternative Communication*. NHS Education for Scotland.

Robinson, H. (2023). The Positive AAC Framework [Poster presentation], Communication Matters Conference, 12 September, 2023.

Teachman, G. and Gibson, B. E. (2014). "Communicative competence" in the field of Augmentative and Alternative Communication: A review and critique. *International Journal of Language & Communication Disorders*, 49(1), 1–14. https://doi.org/10.1111/1460-6984.12055.

PEOPLE

Helen Robinson

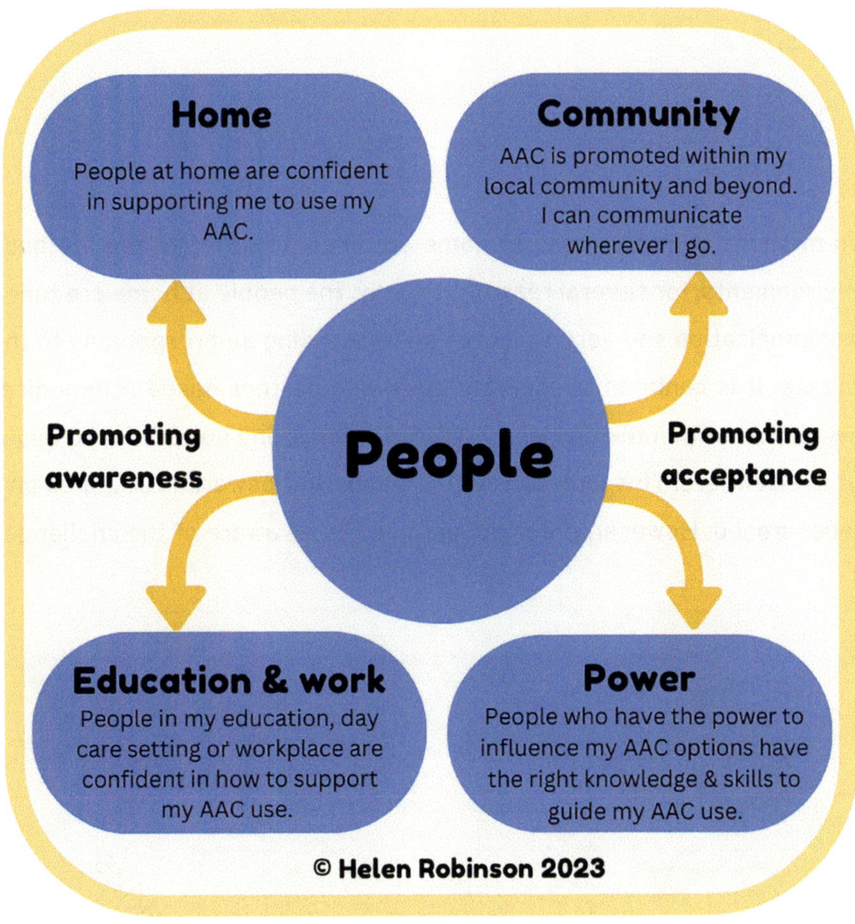
Home
People at home are confident in supporting me to use my AAC.
Community
AAC is promoted within my local community and beyond. I can communicate wherever I go.
Promoting awareness
People
Promoting acceptance
Education & work
People in my education, day care setting or workplace are confident in how to support my AAC use.
Power
People who have the power to influence my AAC options have the right knowledge & skills to guide my AAC use.
© Helen Robinson 2023

Figure 8.1 The People strand from The Positive AAC Framework
Source: Robinson (2023).

The people around an AAC user have great influence over how successful the interaction is. The term "communication partner" is often used. The better skilled the communication partner is, the greater that chance of the AAC user being understood and a connection

DOI: 10.4324/9781003412311-10

made. However, it is important to consider that not every communication partner will need to be equally skilled. Those in regular contact with the AAC user will need to be highly tuned in to their modes of communication, where as those who only encounter the AAC user infrequently will not need to be so skilled, as shown in Jo Holmes and Beth Moulam's communication partner skills map (Holmes and Moulam, 2023), see Figure 8.2.

This chapter focuses on the People strand of The Positive AAC Framework (Robinson, 2023), shown in Figure 8.1. It explores how we can support the people who interact with the AAC user at home, school, the workplace and the community. We will also consider the power that practitioners hold in influencing successful AAC use and the importance of those in privileged positions accessing continued professional development in order to best support AAC users.

Home

The communication methods someone uses at home are likely to differ to the methods they use in other environments, for several reasons. Usually, the people at home are tuned in to the person's communication and very skilled at understanding and responding to the ways they communicate. It is common for person-based and partner-based communication skills to be utilised more within the home environment. Paper and powered AAC might be used less than it is elsewhere. This isn't to say that paper and powered AAC shouldn't be supported and encouraged. However, practitioners need to be aware of the challenges

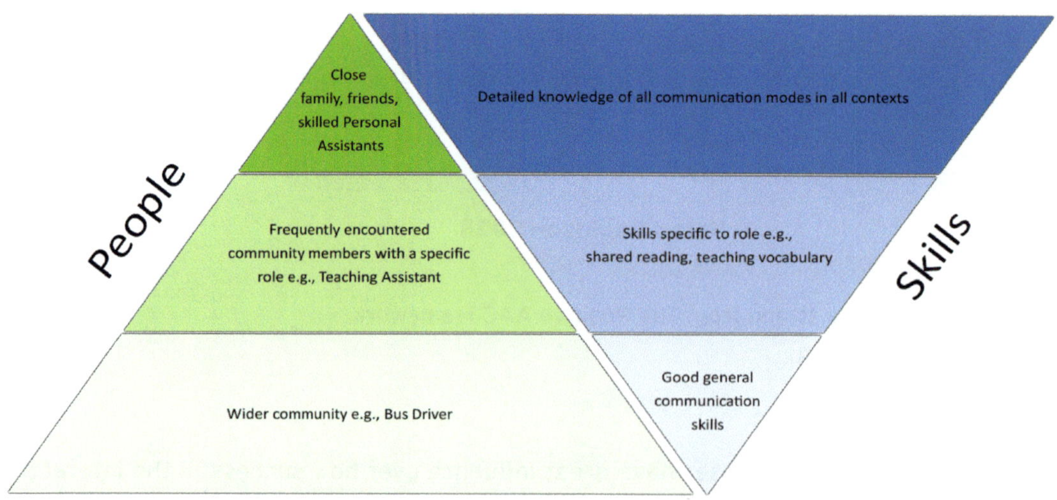

Figure 8.2 Communication partner skills map
Source: Holmes and Moulam (2023).

faced by many families, especially if the AAC user has complex health needs. In Box 8.1, Jo discusses her experiences of using AAC at home with her daughter Lucy.

BOX 8.1 JO DISCUSSES HER EXPERIENCES OF SUPPORTING HER DAUGHTER LUCY'S AAC USE AT HOME

I find times when Lucy's upset or distressed especially difficult. I want to talk to her about her experiences and use AAC but at those times I find it's best to back off with anything language based and connect physically and through tone of voice, in Lucy's case eye contact is helpful. I don't find AAC or symbols support us to co-regulate at all. On a really practical level so much of the support Lucy needs with day-to-day tasks involves both of my hands, personal care, eating and drinking, PEG and medication, hand under hand support, sensory supports and feedback, holding toys and books. For this reason, we rarely use Makaton apart from in songs. It can also be tricky to separate a hand for modelling too. On less of a practical level, more wellbeing, the trauma and exhaustion of the life of parents of children with disabilities is real and well documented. There are times it's just one too many things and nothing happens because my brain is flooded with other things that need doing/we're exhausted from sleepless nights.

At a systemic level I think the way services are delivered mean that professionals are not always able to take full account of the range of challenges for families. For example, there is often a waiting list, we want support but the delay from the time we seek it and the time we get it can mean that a lot has changed. I think we refer to services when we're primed and ready to take something on. By the time we're seen we may have just had a EHCP or a hospital admission or a run of sleepless nights or illness which mean we're not in a place to take on something new. In these contexts, it almost doesn't matter how aware the professionals as they are forced into pathways that don't allow them to be flexible or responsive and timely. I don't believe these decisions are the choice of the therapists on the front line.

I think many of them are "aware". They know it's hard and that there are challenges. Because I've driven much of Lucy's support, I don't know how parents new to this entirely are supported. What I do experience and reflect on is that while I think that individual professionals are "aware", this awareness varies. Something I think professionals need to be aware of is how they use their own experiences to try and demonstrate their awareness. I've had professionals (probably a little more in the early years) talk about their experiences of frustration with communication or eating or drinking in a way that aimed to normalise in a kind of "all kids do that" kind of a way. While this may well be true, I've never found that helpful as it services to feel quite othering. On the other hand, when people have been able to talk about an experience of disability and draw parallels then this has been helpful. For example, when I was taking about feeling frustration and disappointment for lack of funding for a device, one of the therapists we worked with talked briefly about how she had been at odds with services about a wheelchair for her child. This disclosure was brief and did not involve a mass of detail on her part but was enough for me to feel that she had an experience that led to genuine empathy. I think professionals who can't draw on their own experience can also do this by saying things like "I've heard a lot of families feel this way too" or similar.

Joanna Holmes, parent

Understanding the practical and emotional barriers to using AAC at home can help practitioners to offer meaningful support. We must be realistic about what is achievable and understand that for many, having communication aids available and in use continuously is unachievable. As practitioners, we need to be mindful of the feelings of guilt we might perpetuate through the advice we give to families.

In Boxes 8.2, 8.3 and 8.4, two parents of AAC users and an AAC user explain what has helped them use AAC at home.

BOX 8.2 JO SHARES HER ADVICE FOR SEEKING SUPPORT WITH AAC USE

I do like social media for information [but] I think it can easily become overwhelming. I also wonder if the trend to short reels has resulted in entirely helpful media for parents. I see lots of things about modelling all the time, always have the device available etc. which can easily become a pressure to be perfect.

Building AAC support has to work for your family. If it's not working that's OK. Talk to people for support (depending what you need this may be other parents, family members, professionals) until you have a plan that makes you and your family feel good about what you're doing and OK about the things you decide not to do.

Joanna Holmes, parent

BOX 8.3 LISA OFFERS HER ADVICE ON INTRODUCING AAC

Even if the child doesn't take to high-tech AAC or a low tech letterboard straightaway, keep trying ... In terms of teaching AAC, it's important to model and ideally this is done with a second device (£££) but could also be done with printed versions of the symbols or keyboards. If the child doesn't seem to be getting on with a symbol-based system, see how they get on with a keyboard instead. We didn't know my daughter could read or spell until she started writing (supported) and then typing on a keyboard! It's important to teach other family members and friends how to be a good communication partner – things like giving enough time to respond and not talking while the child is typing their message. This is particularly tricky (but important) when video calling.

Lisa Palframan, parent

BOX 8.4 ANDREW (WRITING SUPPORTED BY MELINDA MAYERS) EXPLAINS HOW HE WAS SUPPORTED BY HIS SON TO PERSONALISE HIS COMMUNICATION AID

My son Kai is very techy and he was able to help adding pictures and topics, change set ups, make it more personalised for me. He listened to how I wanted it to look like, what I needed, we tried and tested it together. It is really good because the kids feel involved so it is not so alien for them when I need to use it to say something to them. It became normal through the ways of learning it together.

Andrew Mayers, AAC user

People working with AAC have a duty to support AAC use within the home. We can do this by:

- Taking time to understand the individual circumstances of people's lives.
- Understanding that powered and paper-based AAC might not often be used at home.
- Realising that modelling AAC can be challenging and sometimes become a barrier to co-regulation and connection.
- Aiming to understand the challenges families face, without projecting our own experiences onto them.

Community

We might often think of supporting AAC users in their home or place where they routinely attend, such as a school or adult daycare centre, however, we must remember to think about the wider community in which AAC users live their lives. This includes shopping, travelling, healthcare services, entertainment and leisure. Boxes 8.5, 8.6 and 8.7 provide the experiences of three parents, Jo, Lisa and Lyndsey, regarding their children using AAC in the community:

BOX 8.5 JO DESCRIBES HER EXPERIENCE OF HER DAUGHTER'S AAC USE IN THE COMMUNITY

People are usually either interested (which has its issues in terms of advocacy and how to give info in a short time while not making our lives a training session) or simply accepting. There's one shop in particular in the village where Lucy's chair doesn't fit in the whole shop (and also there are fragile things and she has long sensory seeking arms) so she sits and chats with the owner while I browse. She's become pretty skilled at attributing meaning.

Lucy is a Brownie and her leaders took the time to learn about her communication before she joined. They have seen her transition from Supecore30 with touch access to Coughdrop with larger cells and head tracking and have commented that they have seen an improvement. Her integration at Brownies from an AAC perspective is no doubt helped by the fact that the volunteer who supports her there is an SLT! We also did an AAC awareness session with the Brownies in October and they asked for core boards they could use.

Joanna Holmes, parent

BOX 8.6 LISA DESCRIBES HER EXPERIENCE OF HER DAUGHTER'S AAC USE IN THE COMMUNITY

We've had some positive experiences e.g. patient staff in a restaurant. We were into a sweet shop last week and the lady behind the counter spoke to my wife initially, but when my daughter started using her letterboard (low tech) to make her choices, she addressed my daughter directly. We've been approached by other parents of nonspeaking autistic children when out and about, asking about my daughter and her AAC and how she started communicating. We try to signpost them to useful resources. Less positively, we've had other people speak over my daughter when she's trying to type out her message. She also felt really left out at a big family celebration where we were all sat round the table talking and there was no space for her to speak. When she got upset, her grandmother asked everyone to be quiet and my daughter spoke very eloquently (via her iPad) about how she felt and how people needed to give her the opportunity to join in.

Lisa Palframan, parent

BOX 8.7 LYNDSEY DESCRIBES HER EXPERIENCE OF HER DAUGHTER'S AAC USE IN THE COMMUNITY

It's not something that is familiar to most people. I just don't think it's in people's radar. I also think because we live in a wonderful world of modern technology, we are used to seeing people, especially children with iPads/tablets and I think it could be assumed that a child is playing with a toy rather than using a communication aid.

Lyndsey Hall, parent

Barriers and facilitators to AAC use in the community

Using AAC out and about brings some important practical considerations. People might need to adapt their AAC to suit being away from home or outside. Their powered AAC will need to be loud enough to be heard in crowded, busy environments. People might benefit from the use of a partner screen which displays their message on the outward-facing side of their communication aid, or they might wish to use an amplified case or external Bluetooth speaker. Individuals might opt to take paper-based AAC out with them and leave their powered AAC at home.

Personal safety may be one barrier to AAC use in the community. Having valuable tablet communication aids mounted to a wheelchair can increase a person's vulnerability. We should consider how to ensure the person is as safe as possible, perhaps by ensuring the communication aid is hidden or covered when not in use. For further information on the practical considerations of AAC use see Chapter 7.

Awareness of AAC amongst the general public is increasing, with several media personalities, such as physicist Stephen Hawking and rugby player Rob Burrow, having frequently appeared on our television screens using powered communication aids. In the UK, standup comedian and AAC user Lee Ridley won the television talent contest Britain's Got Talent under his stage name "Lost Voice Guy". There has even been a television sitcom, Speechless (20th Century Fox/ABC Studios), featuring Micah Fowler portraying the character of JJ who uses a laser pointer and letterboard. Box 8.8. gives the perspective of Isabelle Jones, and AAC user on AAC awareness and representation in the media.

BOX 8.8 ISABELLE (WRITING SUPPORTED BY MUM ANNE SIEQUIEN), GIVES HER OPINION ON THE AWARENESS OF AAC WITHIN THE GENERAL PUBLIC

People are so proud when they are wheelchair accessible or have things like induction loops but they haven't learnt yet that lots of people don't speak in the same way and it's not weird, and they should learn to actually listen properly ... lots more needs to be done. Everyone needs to be trained. People should be in films and books using it, and not ones that aren't like real life like Out of My Mind which is American and unrealistic.

Isabelle Jones, AAC user

While the increasing prevalence of AAC use in mainstream media is undoubtedly positive, and leads to a welcome move away from the attitudes Lisa spoke of in box 8.6, where people might presume an AAC user is not capable of contributing, we must also be aware of the potential unrealistic representation of AAC use that the media could portray.

To date, largely the representations of AAC use in the media focus on individuals who are literate and using powered communication aids, communicating using lengthy utterances. We still have a long way to go in terms of portraying a broad range of AAC use and communication difference on our screens. The general public might watch their televisions without knowledge of how the AAC user's message has been composed or delivered. It is likely, especially during interviews, that AAC users will have pre-prepared dialogue that has been scripted and rehearsed with their communication partner, rather than generating and delivering their messages "in the moment". It is understandable that some viewers might perceive communication aids as miraculous mind-reading machines. Beginner AAC users might feel disheartened when their own access method makes message composition frustratingly slow. As practitioners, we can support those we work with by explaining the realities of AAC use on television and offer assurance that they are not failing. We also might wish to consider how we educate our own friends and families about the realities of learning and using AAC, so that if they were to meet an AAC user they would have a more balanced understanding of what is achievable and the effort involved. In Box 8.9, Liz Allen talks about the need for realistic representation of AAC use in the media.

BOX 8.9 LIZ CHAMPIONS THE NEED FOR REALISTIC REPRESENTATIONS OF AAC USE IN THE MEDIA

I would love to see more media about people who communicate in different ways just being normal people getting on with life. I'd also link people to know that AAC isn't a miracle. The chances of putting a device in front of someone and that suddenly they can communicate everything are low. For most people it's a lot of hard work and commitment for small but equally as important gains.

Liz Allen, parent of an AAC user

By increasing the public's awareness of other ways of communicating, we can hope that attitudes towards those with communication differences will improve. In the UK, the Royal College of Speech and Language Therapists has partnered with several charities and organisations, such as the Motor Neurone Disease Association and the Stroke Association, to develop a Communication Access symbol (see Figure 8.3), training package and set of standards, known as CAUK. A free training package is offered to individuals and organisations. Organisations can gain accreditation as Communication Accessible by showing that they demonstrate the standards and can deliver the training. In Box 8.10, AAC user Jill gives her view on the need for communication partner skills training.

BOX 8.10 JILL GIVES HER VIEW ON THE NEED FOR COMMUNICATION PARTNER SKILLS TRAINING

people should learn how to communicate with somebody uses AAC because everyone got right to speak.

Jill Clark, AAC user

The aim of CAUK is to train employees of businesses and organisations to be confident in engaging with people who have communication difficulties and differences. Businesses and organisations which have gained accreditation can display the Communication Access symbol which lets customers and service users know that their staff will be supportive of their ways of communicating (Communication Access UK, n.d.).

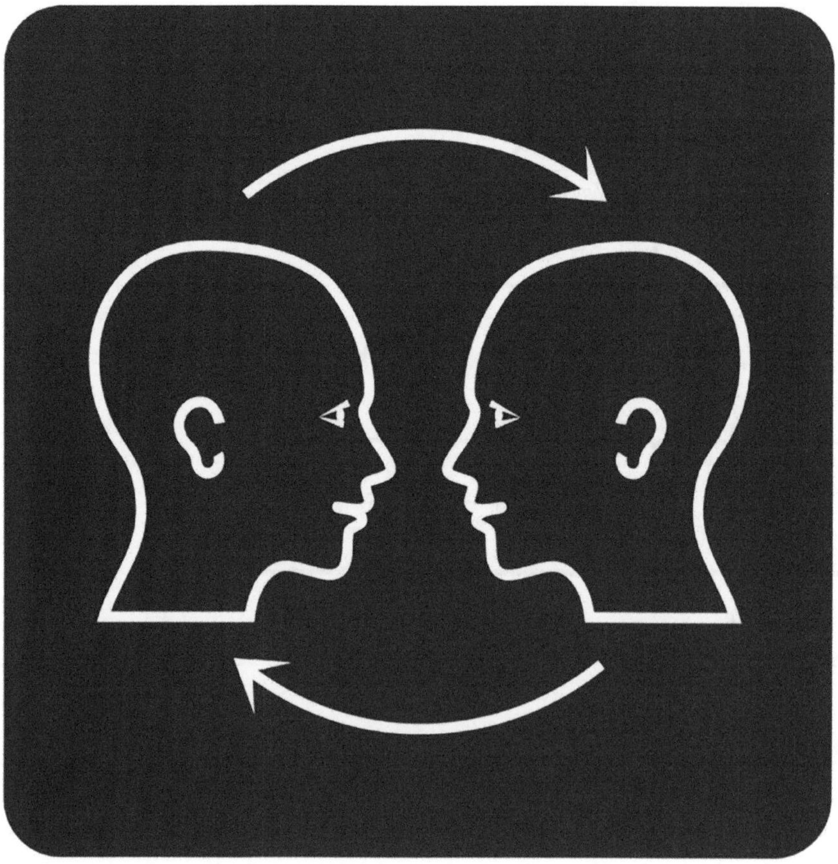

Figure 8.3 The Communication Access Symbol for the UK
Source: Communication Access UK (nd).

People working with AAC have a duty to promote awareness of AAC beyond the AAC user's immediate environment. We can do this by:

- Talking about AAC with our own friends and family.
- Volunteering our time for community groups, such as Scout groups, to raise awareness of AAC.
- Promoting training and awareness raising programmes, such as the CAUK accreditation.

Education, adult daycare and work

Individuals might spend the majority of their daytime hours away from home, perhaps at school, work or attending an adult day care setting, among other places. The people in these settings therefore have great power in facilitating AAC use and require support in understanding how they might do this.

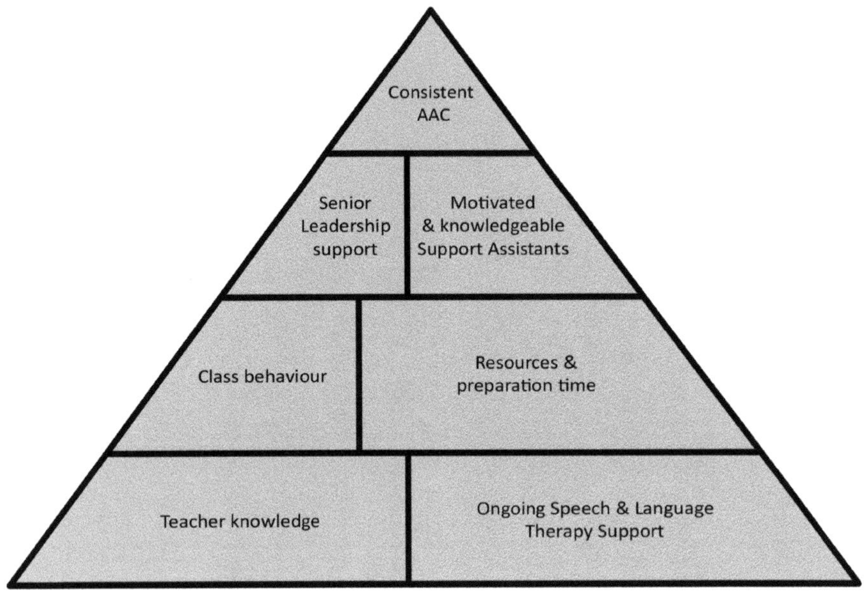

Figure 8.4 Nature of the beast
Source: Doran (2023).

Education settings

Supporting effective AAC use in educational settings can be challenging, both for the practitioners in the classroom and external practitioners and families. AAC use is a small part of what happens during a typical day in a classroom. Figure 8.4 shows what needs to be in place for consistent AAC use to occur, according to Joseph Doran, who is a teacher with experience of supporting AAC.

The challenges faced in relation to each of the sub-sections from Figure 8.4 will be considered here:

Teacher knowledge

Often, teachers are given minimal teaching in communication difficulties and differences. While there are undoubtedly many teachers with expertise, many will not have taught an AAC user before, especially if it is a mainstream educational setting.

On-going SLT support

In the UK, many speech and language therapists work to a consultative model, where they have minimal direct interaction with the AAC user themselves. This means that the responsibility of implementing AAC often falls to the adults in the classrooms. There will also be schools who have no input from a speech and language therapist. Where SLTs do have designated one-to-one time with pupils, this can mean that education practitioners think that the AAC work has been taken care of and doesn't require further support.

Class behaviour

Teachers and classroom assistants will be managing classroom behaviour constantly, which can mean AAC implementation isn't prioritised. Adults in the classroom will be managing the needed of many children, not just the AAC users.

Resources and prep time

AAC implementation will require some level of forward planning, whether it's printing off symbols or photographs, recording messages into a communication aid or adding new vocabulary. Education practitioners are unlikely to be given designated time to do this. There will also be additional skills required to do this work, such as knowing how to use graphic symbol software or how to edit vocabulary.

Motivated and knowledgeable learning support assistants

AAC users will often be directly supported by learning support assistants/teaching assistants. Having them on-board with AAC use is important. To do this, they will need to understand what AAC is and why it is important.

Senior leadership support

Ultimately, the senior leadership team within a school will influence policy and practice. Having a leadership team that both understands what AAC is and places appropriate value on it is vital. Working with the leadership team to develop their knowledge of AAC will have benefits that cascade throughout the school.

Familiar challenges

The hope of many AAC practitioners is that their specialist input will lead to better AAC in the classroom and as illustrated in Figure 8.5, there are several barriers to achieving this:

- Lack of knowledge
- Resistance to change
- Lack of time for training

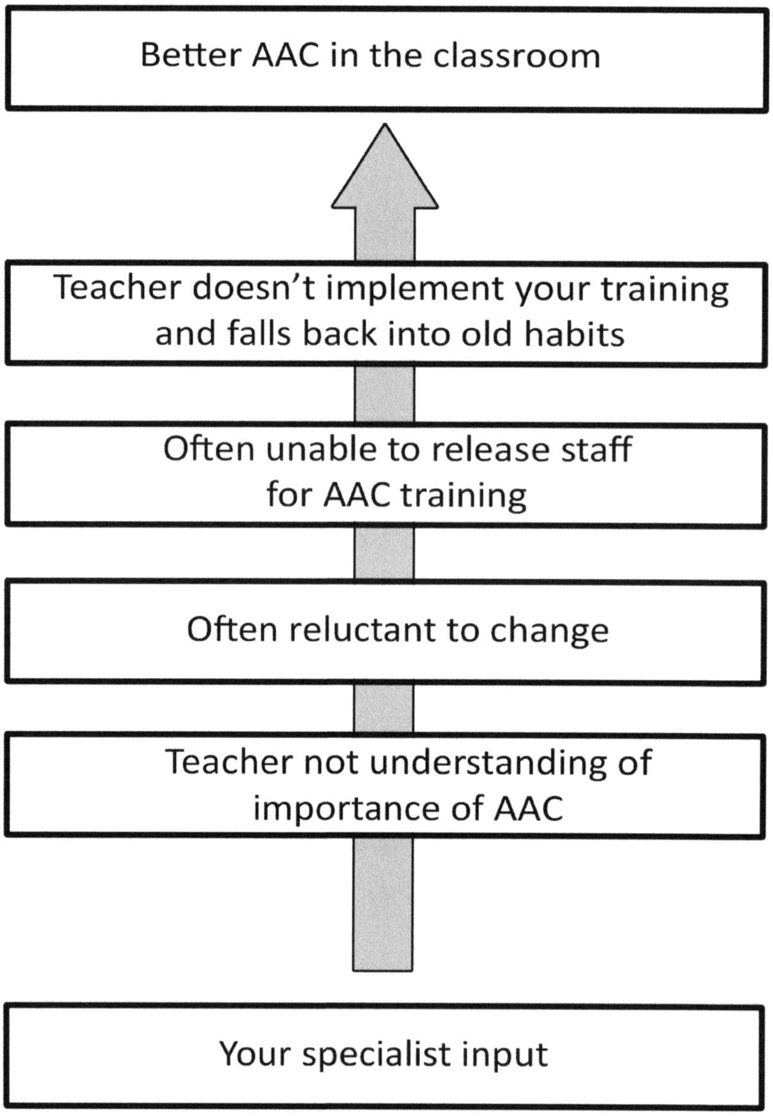

Figure 8.5 Nature of the beast part 2: revenge of the beast
Source: Doran (2023).

How to develop people's knowledge

Focus on getting people to practice what you're teaching them. Describing how to do something usually isn't enough, show them and then get them to show you. Give people a little bit of research and theory, but don't fall into the trap of trying to teach them everything you know, or trying to justify your advice. Keep it simple and practical.

How to support resistance to change

Invite collaboration by asking the teacher what they would like the AAC user to achieve. This might not perfectly align with what you are thinking and it could be way off, but use this as a starting point and work from there.

Plan a time for discussion, outside of the classroom if possible. Handing over a page of targets and/or advice is unlikely to be well received. Discussing targets or giving advice while the teacher is teaching is not going to be effective.

How to affect change when time is limited

Understand that the AAC user you are supporting is one of a (potentially large) group of young people. They may be the only AAC user, or one of many who are using different modes of AAC. It is important to look for quick wins, considering what can the education practitioners easily achieve. The aim is to convince education practitioners that following your advice will make their life easier! Advice should be linked to specific daily activities within the classroom. Aim to make it clear, applicable and part of the routine. Ask people to make suggestions and think of ideas themselves and be prepared to challenge where necessary.

Other settings

Other settings might include (but are not limited to) adult daycare, respite, hospital and rehabilitation centres and places of work. A particular challenge in settings such as these is the large number of people coming into contact with the AAC user. Beyond education, it is less likely that the AAC user will have one person dedicated to supporting them, and therefore providing effective training becomes a greater challenge.

In education, we might be able to gather the team working with the child in one place to deliver training, but gathering all the healthcare staff in a rehabilitation unit or hospital ward is very unlikely. We must therefore adapt how we support the AAC user in these settings. The templates *Communication aid set-up guide*, *Communication aid support plan* and *How to help me communicate*, found in Chapter 7, can be useful in settings such as this.

In Box 8.11, speech and language therapist Alison talks about the barriers of AAC use for children outside of home and school.

BOX 8.11 ALISON TALKS ABOUT THE BARRIERS OF AAC USE FOR CHILDREN OUTSIDE OF HOME AND SCHOOL

Often when a child is admitted with an acute illness the communication aid stays at home or in school so they are then in a strange environment without their usual form of communication. This can also happen in going to respite or any other environment. Even in outpatient appointments the child often does not have their communication aid with them and the family need to be reminded to bring it so the child can be assessed or at least contribute to the conversation. Part of this can be about who paid for the device – if school have paid for the device or it belongs to school then it tends to stay there and makes it difficult to access when the child has a long stay in hospital – or is anywhere outside of school. I firmly believe that if a child has a device, it should be used as their own voice and should not be only available to them in one setting which is only one part of their life. Also, both low tech and high-tech supports can be put away in cupboards because of change-over staff and they don't know what it's for and put it to one side. Or people are intimidated by using it.

It can take some time to learn how to use the system and the whole process can be quite time consuming. It's often as much about the carer learning the system as the child learning to use it. It's new to everyone – especially in an acute acquired setting. It's a completely new way of interacting. Or they can see it as the SLTs "task of the day" rather than something which needs to go on routinely.

Alison Felton, speech and language therapist

Training

There are different formats that training people to support AAC might take, including:

- Group training sessions, e.g. school teams, adult daycare staff.
- One-to-one training sessions e.g. parent, spouse or key worker.
- Online resources e.g. webinars, e-learning packages, websites, social media content.
- Handouts/information sheets and leaflets.

We will need to adapt the method we use to deliver information according to the existing skills and knowledge of those supporting the AAC user and the logistics of the setting. We should consider:

- What experience of AAC do people already have?
- Is it possible to gather everyone together?
- Would one-to-one training be more appropriate?
- How do people prefer to learn?

Where possible, we should involve the AAC user themselves in delivering the training, both in the planning of the content and the delivery. If this isn't possible, then consider using others with lived experience in your training and resources.

A guide for topics to cover in AAC training is provided here:

- About the person:
  - Describe their communication skills and preferences.
  - Describe their AAC experience.
- About the AAC:
  - What's the name of the AAC (e.g. iPad, PODD book, Big Mack), what's the name of the software and vocabulary (e.g. Grid 3 and Super Core) and what will you all call it (e.g. talker, communication aid, symbol book)?
  - How does the person access the AAC (e.g. head mouse, finger, eye pointing)?
  - How to operate and use the AAC if it is powered (charging, on/off, volume, mounting).
- Operating the software (if using). To include: access settings, pronunciation exceptions, backing up the user profile, editing the vocabulary.
- Navigating the vocabulary:
  - How is the language organised?
  - What is the theory behind the organisation (e.g. core vocabulary, pragmatic organisation, visual scenes, gestalts)?
- Implementing/supporting the AAC use:
  - How to model AAC use (see Chapter 6).
  - What to do if the AAC isn't working or people need further support.
- Goal setting
  - What are the current goals for AAC?
  - What is the plan to support this (who, what, when) and when will it be reviewed?

If training isn't possible, for example, in a hospital ward where staff cannot all be available, then we need to ensure accessible information is clearly visible to those coming into contact with the AAC user, by keeping user-guides and helpful information with the communication aid or near to the person (e.g., on the wall next to their hospital bed).

Barriers and facilitators

It can be helpful to consider the barriers and facilitators which impact successful AAC use within each setting and also between the many dyads (pairs of people), such as AAC and their spouse, the AAC users and their teacher or the AAC user and their friend. Barriers and facilitators might be within the areas of knowledge, skills and attitudes of each person, or groups of people (Beeke and Bloch, 2023; Da Fonte and Boesch, 2018).

Sometimes, people might be comfortable to say they don't have the necessary skills to support AAC, they might even be able to name specific areas they need help with. Often, people will be reluctant to admit they are lacking in skills, or will simply be unaware of the knowledge they don't have. This can make it a challenge for practitioners to know what support is required. Discussion with individuals and teams, alongside observation, can be useful ways of identifying the barriers and facilitators.

The Better Conversations therapy approach (Beeke and Bloch, 2023) uses observations of the AAC user and their partner (which may be recorded) to enable the speech and language therapist to identify the barriers and facilitators within a conversation. The approach then supports both conversation partners to set goals around skills and barriers, using their preferred strategies. See Beeke and Bloch (2023) for further information on this approach.

Power

Those of us privileged to work with AAC users must recognise the power we hold in influencing their AAC journey. It is our responsibility to ensure we have the appropriate knowledge and skills to offer quality assessment, solutions and support. We might ask ourselves the following questions:

- Am I getting my knowledge from a range of sources, including those with lived experience, peer networks, AAC product vendors, conferences, online sources and peer-reviewed journals?
- Am I willing to change my practice and consider new ways of working?
- Am I sharing my knowledge and learning? Either within my immediate team, wider peer networks or via social media?
- Am I willing to challenge others who may be using outdated theory and practice?

Some helpful ways to keep up to date with current practice are given here:

- **Social media accounts.** Look for those with lived experience of AAC and the people that support them. AAC practitioners and product vendors are also useful accounts to follow.
- **AAC blogs.** Subscribing to AAC blogs will ensure regular updates of current AAC theory and practice.
- **Training offered by AAC product vendors.** Most AAC product vendors will offer regular online or in-person training, often free of charge.

- **AAC Networks.** There are a range of networks offering peer support and regular in-person or online meet ups. There will usually be guest speakers and the opportunity to learn about current theory and practice. Consider looking for or setting up local per support groups in your area too.
- **Peer-reviewed journals.** These provide current research, but can be challenging to access free of charge. Some authors publish open access papers, so it's worth following AAC researchers on social media to be informed of new publications.

When seeking knowledge, we must question the information we are consuming and view it with a critical lens. Some key questions to ask ourselves are:

- Who is this information coming from? What motives might they have (e.g., selling a product or service)? What is the source of this message?
- Is this information supportive of different ways of communicating or does it perpetuate an ableist viewpoints of communication?

Summary

Supporting the people around the AAC user is often a challenging process and dependent on many variables. It is therefore difficult to have a template for how to support AAC implementation, and the practitioner will need to respond flexibly to each situation.

It is important that practitioners recognise the power they hold in directing a person's AAC journey and therefore make the effort to keep themselves informed of ever-changing theory and practice, via a range of sources.

References

Beeke, S. and Bloch, S. (eds) (2023). *Better Conversations with Communication Difficulties: A Practical Guide for Clinicians*. J & R Press Ltd.

Communication Access UK. (nd). The Communication Access Symbol for the UK. https://communication-access.co.uk/about/.

Da Fonte, M. A. and Boesch, M. C. (2018). *Effective Augmentative and Alternative Communication Practices: A Handbook for School-based Practitioners*. Routledge.

Doran, J. (2023, September 10). Talking to Teachers: Guidance for Speech and Language Therapists working with Teachers to implement better AAC [Conference presentation]. Communication Matters Conference, Leeds University, United Kingdom.

Holmes, J. and Moulam, B. (2023, September 10). Communication Partner Skills [Conference presentation]. Communication Matters Conference, Leeds University, United Kingdom.

Robinson, H. (2023, December 9). The Positive AAC Framework [Poster presentation]. Communication Matters Conference, Leeds University of Leeds, UK.

9

PRIDE

Helen Robinson

The pride movement is associated with groups of marginalised people, in particular the LGBTQIA+ community (e.g., gay pride and transgender pride). While the LGBTQIA+ pride movement originated over 50 years ago, the disability pride movement is comparatively

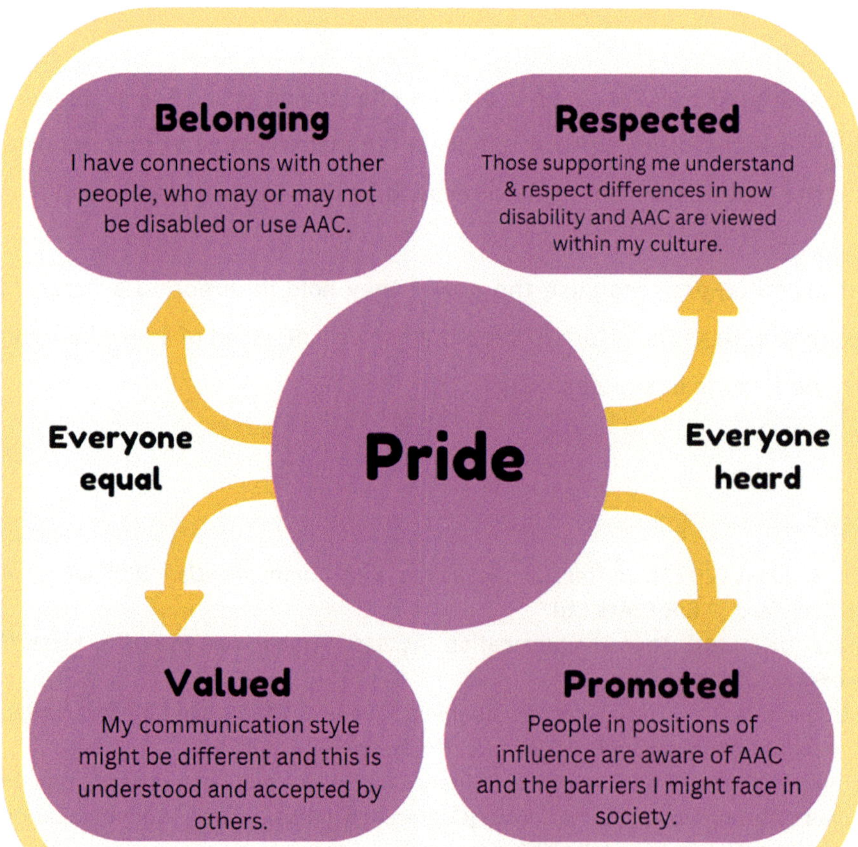

Belonging
I have connections with other people, who may or may not be disabled or use AAC.
Respected
Those supporting me understand & respect differences in how disability and AAC are viewed within my culture.
Everyone equal
Pride
Everyone heard
Valued
My communication style might be different and this is understood and accepted by others.
Promoted
People in positions of influence are aware of AAC and the barriers I might face in society.
© Helen Robinson, 2023

Figure 9.1 The Pride strand from The Positive AAC Framework
Source: Robinson (2023).

DOI: 10.4324/9781003412311-11

new and relatively unknown. Rooted in the 1990 Americans with Disabilities Act (ADA), the social model of disability and the Disability Rights Movement, and making its way into UK society in 2015. Pride is both a celebration of identity but also a way to raise awareness and protest against stigmatisation, discrimination and oppression (Bogart, Lund and Rottenstein, 2018).

Stigma is the negative attitudes within society associated with the mental, physical or social characteristics of individuals or groups. Stigmatisation is closely linked to low self-esteem, the impact of which can be lessened by people joining together. Challenging dominant beliefs of disability as something negative, disability pride "views disability as a source of valuable, enriching and positive experience" (Bogart, Lund and Rottenstein, 2018, p. 155) and can reduce the negative effects of stigma. Pride encourages a shift in the narrative of disability as something to be ashamed of or pitied, to one where it is celebrated as part of human diversity (Niedbalski, 2023). Therefore, it is important to consider how those working with AAC users can support individuals to develop a sense of pride and recognise the barriers to doing so.

Belonging

The popular terminology of "Equality, Diversity and Inclusion" (EDI) is beginning to be replaced by "Equity, Diversity and Belonging" (EDB) or "Diversity, Equity, Inclusion and Belonging" (DEIB). Whereas the term equality was previously used to ensure everybody was treated the same, the term equity refers to the fair treatment of individuals based on their specific needs and circumstances.

Diversity refers to the variation in human differences, such as gender, race and sexual orientation. Inclusion is often used to mean that an individual's diversity is respected to allow them to participate in society. Those who are viewed as "different" to the societal norm are often met with fear and discrimination. Social exclusion is associated with segregation and the placement of those with differences away from mainstream society. Those belonging to marginalised groups, including people with communication difficulties and differences, are seen as "other". It is this "otherness" that creates a sense of not belonging; to be excluded from society is not to belong (Hall, 2010; Kewanian, Creely and Southcott, 2024).

A Facebook post from Jo Holmes in Box 9.1 discusses her thoughts, as a parent of an AAC user, on inclusion regarding a news story reporting on the removal of a disabled child from a class photograph.

BOX 9.1 JO HOLMES, MUMMY VS AAC FACEBOOK POST (29 MARCH 2024)

I feel so curious about why somebody would make the decision to offer a picture that didn't have a child with complex needs in it when that child is part of the class. And it's really got me thinking what sort process did the photographer or the person who makes the decision about how pictures will be presented was thinking about when they made that decision to have an option what removed a child with disabilities from the picture. I wonder if it's a decision about symmetry.

I think we're all familiar with the traditional image of a school photograph children in line some sat on benches. Some stood on benches, and some stood in between with the teacher at end of the row. I wonder if the presence of a child, maybe a big wheelchair with tubes and medical equipment, upset the symmetry.

But the thing is for our children to be really present in our communities and in our towns and cities and villages and schools and places of worship and shops and playgrounds, we need to be prepared to sacrifice the tidiness of symmetry.

I believe that, almost everyone, if you ask them would want to live in a more inclusive society. Still though disabled children and their families live in a world that is not built and organised for us. For that to happen, everybody needs to think about creating communities, built environments and education systems that make and leave space for everyone.

The challenge is (it) upsets the symmetry ...

... it means accepting that access to toilets costs money.

... it means that it's OK for there to be loads of empty blue badge spaces because they're there if someone who needs them needs them.

... it means a society that allows extra space in conversations for people who need more time to be heard and understood.

... it means EVERYONE accepting that to build a society that's really inclusive means accepting the asymmetry, doing the work, not just on physical spaces but attitude too.

... it's means letting our children take up space... even if it upsets the symmetry.

Joanna Holmes, parent

Social exclusion can be attributed to structures, institutions and sociocultural causes, or it can be viewed as the responsibility of the individual and place the focus on what they must do to make themselves more included in society. Rather than looking at how society has failed to include disabled people, the blame is placed on the person themselves. The expectation is that individuals will take steps to participate in society by becoming more "normal" instead of looking at how society might change in order to include everyone. More specifically within the field of AAC, successful inclusion might be attributed to the technology rather than the user, whereas perceived "failure" to use AAC (and be included) might be blamed on the person themselves being unmotivated or incapable (Sellwood et al., 2024).

There is a tendency to link successful inclusion to the contribution a person makes to society, which is often assessed via employment, independent living and community participation (Chapman, 2023; Hall, 2010), however, belonging is much more than being included in mainstream spaces. Disabled people may be given opportunities for paid employment for example, but this does not automatically mean they will feel like they belong (Scorgie, with Forlin, 2019).

Hall (2010) states that "To belong is to feel attached, to feel valued, and to have a sense of insiderness and proximity to 'majority' people, activities, networks and spaces" (Hall, 2010, p. 56). Scorgie and Forlin (2019) offer a further definition:

> Social inclusion incorporates attitudes, expectations and perceptions about what it means to belong to a group. Belonging is embedded in personal beliefs and social structures that set forth criteria that determine how individuals and groups and accorded value and esteem.
>
> *(Scorgie and Forlin, 2019, p. 3)*

To not belong has significant consequences to an individual's sense of well-being and mental health; it is a fundamental human need to belong. There is societal pressure to change and adapt oneself in order to conform and therefore belong, and to be different is seen a deficit.

Over recent years, there has been a move away from a deficit-based model towards a strengths- and abilities-based approach. The challenges of embracing a person-centred, strengths-based approach within educational and wider societal structures that focus on measurement, developmental norms and comparison has been widely observed (Brea-Spahn and Bauler, 2023; Cushing, 2022; Kewanian, Creely and Southcott, 2024; Nair, Farah and Cushing, 2023).

A sense of belonging, and therefore pride, might be achieved through interactions who have shared lived experiences. Connecting with others who share characteristics and face similar challenges can foster a sense of belonging. AAC users might have a lot to gain through meeting other AAC users, including access to role models who might inspire and empower.

The likelihood of individuals identifying as disabled and seeking out others like them is dependent on the degree of their impairment, their age, ethnicity, income and experience of stigma. Those born with developmental conditions may be more likely to identify as disabled than those with acquired conditions who may experience a loss of identity following the onset of their condition and struggle to identify as a disabled person and seek out new communities (Bogart, 2017).

Individuals might also seek belonging through interactions with those who share similar interests and hobbies. People have the right to exclude themselves from groups as well as be included. AAC users may not wish to seek out other AAC users; what matters is sense of agency and choice over the connections that are available to an individual. Often, the idea of where a disabled person might "belong" is decided by non-disabled practitioners, perpetuating ableist viewpoints (Scorgie, with Forlin, 2019; Shew, 2023).

BOX 9.2 SIMON DESCRIBES HOW HIS COMMUNICATION AID SUPPORTS HIM TO FEEL INCLUDED

My name is Simon and I am 55 years old. I have FND *(functional neurological disorder)* and on the 7th of October 2023 my voice left me. My life was turned upside down. I didn't realise how much we took for granted our speech. It was more difficult for me because I also loose the use of my upper body, so a lot of the time I wasn't able to write things down or use an app on my phone that speaks for you.

I got a speech therapist involved and she put me forward for an AAC Machine. A machine I have never heard of before. I was going to be able to speak with my eyes. This sounded too good to be true. For the next couple of months, I had alphabet cards to spell out words to form sentences and picture cards for things that I wanted with the help of the wife but it was a nightmare.

Then late December the AAC machine arrived. I got the hang of it straight way. It is the most amazing thing. I felt like I had got my life back. When I am sat in a paralysed state, I can still take part in conversations. When we have friends round, I can make conversation and even have a laugh with the symoji.

For those first couple of months my wife wouldn't leave me alone but because I can WhatsApp or Email from the machine, I can keep in touch with her or she can keep in touch with me.

I can also control the TV when I am on own so I can be left. The machine has given me independence and also my wife some freedom. I felt so afraid at times without my voice as I was always a big talker but the AAC gave me hope and gave me, my new normal life back. They are amazing.

Simon Snell, AAC user

To support AAC users to develop connections with others and embody a sense of belonging, practitioners may reflect on the following questions:

- To what extent do I engage AAC users and their families in decision making?
- How do I support AAC users to find their community?
- Am I signposting AAC users to sources of mentorship, advocacy and role models?
- What am I doing to promote the voices of those I work with, giving them opportunities to be heard?

Respected

In order to promote equity, diversity and belonging, practitioners must respect the cultural background of each individual and how that may impact on their experience of using AAC (Pope, Light and Franklin, 2022). Omino and Negesh (2023) define culture as "the systems of knowledge shared by a relatively large group of people. Cultural factors are more related to religion, ethnicity and tradition" (p. 565). Culture may influence whether or not a person identifies as disabled, whether they access support and if they might engage with activism. Pride has been shown to be associated with those who are White, young and independent (Bogart, Lund and Rottenstein, 2018).

Ableism refers to the discrimination of people based on their disability and is closely linked with racism and white supremacy (Shew, 2023). Some labels and terminology intended to empower disabled people within the Global West can actually be problematic for some people from Black and Minority Ethnic (BAME) backgrounds, leading to further marginalisation. The word disabled itself can be an issue (Harvey and Charles, 2023).

Julie Charles is a Black disabled woman born in London with Dominican and Aruban heritage. She discusses the differing approaches of these three cultures to disability. "Labels can misrepresent and deny identity as much as they can be used to create community and unity" (Harvey and Charles, 2023, p. 89). People may not identify as being a disabled person and to be described as such can feel embarrassing.

Charles talks about the word "handicapped" still being familiar in her culture, whereas it would be seen as offensive to many people from the Global West. Many languages don't have the word "disabled" or even the concept as understood by Western cultures. Other cultures might name the illness, condition or mental state, and see disability as "a white person thing" (Harvey and Charles, p. 90).

Viewing their difficulties and differences through a non-western lens can mean that people from BAME backgrounds might not be comfortable accessing services if living in the Global West. Use of the term "disabled" by practitioners might cause offence and to exist in the Western world might mean that people from BAME communities are forced into identifying as disabled, despite the repercussions for themselves and their families, so that they might access the support they require. This could be viewed as colonialism (Harvey and Charles, 2023) where linguistic hierarchies are placed on those from BAME backgrounds, forcing them to take on the Westernised terminology and conceptualisation of disability which might not fit with that of their own culture: "Accepting the label is accepting the white man's label for how we should understand ourselves. Like we had to in slavery. In colonies" (Harvey and Charles, 2023, p. 94).

Those working with AAC users must understand the importance of intersectionality. This refers to a person belonging to two or more marginalised groups, for example: being Black and being transgender. Intersectionality creates a unique experience of AAC use for each person and it is therefore important for practitioners to be considerate of the different marginalised groups to which a person may belong. There is a growing body of literature highlighting the prevalence of racism, white supremacy and colonialism within speech and language therapy (Brea-Spahn and Bauler, 2023; Cushing, 2022; Nair, Farah and Cushing, 2023; Pope, Light and Franklin, 2022; Yu, Epstein and Tisi, 2021).

Huer (2000) found differences in the way graphic symbols are interpreted by people from different cultural backgrounds and suggests that differing linguistic and life experiences will influence symbol interpretation. Practitioners therefore need to be mindful of this when selecting graphic symbols and ensure that the AAC users and/or their families are included in symbol choice.

Pope, Light and Franklin (2022) compared the level of AAC intervention received by Black children with that received by White children and found that Black children were significantly disadvantaged. As well as receiving less AAC support than their White peers, Black and Asian children with developmental delay are less likely to receives a diagnosis, or receive one later in childhood. The concerns of Black and Asian children's parents are more likely to be ignored. Pope, Light and Franklin (2022) also highlighted that most AAC research is conducted with White children and is not representative of BAME communities and further research into equitable service delivery is required. While the reasons for the disparity in AAC service delivery are unclear, the attitudes and beliefs of those supporting AAC users may be contributing, for example, having low expectations of parental support and therefore providing less therapeutic intervention. Practitioners are encouraged to engage in self-reflection and examine racial disparity within their caseloads and wider service delivery. Identifying barriers and solutions needs to use a collaborative approach across services as well as including families and AAC users in the planning of AAC support.

In order to demonstrate understanding and respect for cultural differences and the impact on AAC use, practitioners may reflect on the following questions:

- To what extent is my practice influenced by my implicit bias (e.g. attitudes toward race, gender, sexuality and socioeconomic status).
- What steps am I taking to educate myself about the cultural differences of those I support?
- To what extent is the way I work dominated by ideologies that favour the White, middle-class, Global Western viewpoint?
- Am I continually engaging in acts of anti-racism?
- What am I doing to name and disrupt policy and practice which is harmful to marginalised groups?

Valued

The use of standardised testing is commonplace within speech and language therapy. These standardised ideologies of what is "normal" or "appropriate" communication underpin many of the care pathways and support plans used today. The developmental norms against which individuals are judged are rooted in colonialism, being developed and imposed by the White middle class. These norms marginalise and exclude individuals who communicate in ways deemed to be non-standard. Speech and language therapy practices are still often rooted in the medical model, with the aim to "fix" and "cure", viewing spoken communication as better than other modalities (Brea-Spahn and Bauler, 2023).

Ableism and racism feature heavily in Western society (Nair, Farah and Cushing, 2023; Yu, Epstein and Tisi, 2021) and capitalism continues to be an overbearing influence on the way communication differences are viewed. A person's value is often based on their ability to contribute to society (Shew, 2023). Joncour writes: "The value of a human being is massively based on their capacity to correspond to norms: productivity, verbal communication, having a standardized body and behaviour, showing the power of their physical and mental strength" (Joncour, 2023, p. 130).

Value judgements are placed on the mode of communication a person uses, their literacy skills, their vocabulary use, articulation abilities and ability to perform according to perceived rules of social interaction.

Andrea Lee, Speech and Language Therapist for the Barnsley Assistive Technology Team, writes about the importance of valuing the varying ways in which communicative functions might be expressed by AAC users:

Communicative functions

Communicative functions are categories which are used to break down and analyse parts of conversations. There is no one definitive list of communicative functions but the lists commonly used often include categories such as greetings, requesting, comments, provision of information, protesting, clarification and more. Different communicative actions can be defined as having different functions. For example, a wave may be defined as a "greeting", a point towards an object may be a "request", a spoken phrase may "provide information" (Clarke and Kirton 2003; Pennington and McConachie 1999;).

While these familiar lists are predominantly formed from typical communication styles of speaking individuals, there have been recent shifts to considering wider inclusion of atypical communicative functions, particularly those seen in autistic communication styles. For example, more recent lists may describe functions as "self" or "other"; "self" functions may include internal dialogue or sensory or interest based regulatory functions whereas "other" may refer to those used to connect socially with others (Beverly Vicker, M.S., CCC-SLP, n.d.).

Communicative functions were originally developed for use in research as a means of describing and comparing conversational styles. Within AAC research, they have been used to show conversational patterns (Clarke and Kirton, 2003; Pennington and Mcconachie, 1999) which can then be used to inform clinical practice.

While the assessment of a person's communicative functions can be a very useful descriptive measure, there are times when this may not be appropriate or may need to be used flexibly. Communication functions are based on the notion that there are typical features which make up most conversations. It is important that this notion is not applied in a way that pathologises or devalues atypical features or enforces typical features.

AAC users may use communicative functions differently to speaking communicators due to the need to integrate their communication aid and their multimodal communication. It can be very effortful and slow for AAC users to find all the words they need so they may choose to communicate several functions with one communicative action and have these differentiated by the partner clarifying. For example, they may choose to use looking at the clock for the three very different functions of requesting information: "What time is it?", giving information: "It's time to go" or expressing emotion: "You're late". These individual differences in how communicative functions are expressed should be encouraged as they demonstrate and can help to develop strategic and social communication skills.

Some communicators may have a style where they show a preference towards certain functions and don't naturally use others. This is often seen in autistic communicators who may find provision of information suits their style more than greetings or requesting information. The broad spectrum of communication function profiles is representative of the neurodiverse population and AAC users should be encouraged to use the functions that work for them.

Some clinical assessment or goal setting tools have adopted lists of communicative functions as a means of capturing how an AAC user is using their communication aid. This can provide useful information which can then be used for measuring progress, setting goals, sharing information and building a communicative profile. Two widely used tools which use communicative functions are C.O.D.E.S. (The Keycomm Team, 2011) and the Pragmatics Profile for AAC (Martin, Small and Stevens, 2017). These tools are particularly useful for discussion in training when an AAC user and their team may have got stuck communicating or modelling one particular function, such as "requesting", and may want to broaden their range to explore different functions.

While for the most part, the assessment of an AAC user's communicative functions is clinically beneficial, there is the potential for misuse which should be considered. The interpretation of communicative functions may be detrimental, not neurodiverse affirming, or ableist when used for the following purposes.

- To grade a person's communication style. Both the Pragmatics Profile and C.O.D.E.S. clearly state that they are not intended for this.
- To measure one person's communication against another's, against a perceived gold standard or against normative functions.
- To compare atypical communication styles against typical communication styles.
- To standardise an individual's communication style, that is, to impose a function that is not natural to the person or try to "fix" an atypical function.
- To pathologise or devalue atypical communicative functions or those not listed in the tools. Functions which may not feature on the standard lists are often seen in autistic communicators, for example, self-talk, echolalia, self-regulation talk or self-stimulatory talk (stimming).
- When personal value judgements by clinician/adult/speaker are imposed on the AAC user. Someone with no religious beliefs could be tempted to make a judgement on the communicative function of solitary or communal prayer or a non-autistic person may be tempted to make a judgement on the importance of using greetings. An awareness of internal bias needs to be carefully considered when thinking about another person's use of communicative functions.

Communicative functions are a feature, and not the entirety, of an interaction. It is essential that communicative functions are viewed in context and do not become the end goal of an intervention. The impact of an interaction may be more significant than the functions used. For example, a young child may ask a question repeatedly with the primary function being to practice initiating, an autistic person may repeatedly ask a question to request reassurance and a person with dementia may ask a question repeatedly but with the function of maintaining a "safe", familiar interaction. None of these situations may actually be using the repeated questioning for the function of "requesting information".

Consequently, communicative functions observed should always be contextualised with the modes of communication, the partners and the environment. If we consider the overall purposes of communication as being to belong, to create social connections and to interact comfortably with our environment then we can observe much richer functions than just those conveyed in the message content. Interactions such as those where the engagement is through shared humour, offering comfort, creating a momentary connection or through reciprocity such as a shared song, are some of the most impactful interactions but are often the most difficult to capture through the analysis of functions alone.

(*With thanks to Andrea Lee for providing her thoughts on communicative functions.*)

What can we do to promote societal acceptance of different ways of communicating?

The Disability Pride movement has demonstrated several positive outcomes gained from "coming out" as disabled. Being out and open about one's disability can enable individuals to find others like them, seek out allies to support them, change societal views of their disability and increase representation in the media. This in turn may reduce the level of stigma faced by disabled people (Bogart, Lund and Rottenstein, 2018).

We can begin to value the diversity in communication styles by first accepting the natural diversity in the use of communication modalities, communicative functions and utterance length. Often, the emphasis is placed on assessing a person's differences compared to societal norms. It is often assumed that normalisation is the ultimate goal (Shew, 2023). Practitioners are instead encouraged to shift their focus towards development strengths-based support plans.

The use of Patient Reported Outcome Measures (PROMS) is not yet widely in place but would serve as a more individually centred way of planning support, rather than developmental norms and checklists which are currently in use (see Chapter 7).

Research into AAC design needs to be user-led and focus on the communication needs and styles of AAC users. Currently, AAC design is driven by mainstream technologies which are built around ableist values and assumptions as to what is appropriate or required. Sellwood et al. (2024) propose a manifesto for AAC design in which they

> 1. question the dominance of predictions that artificial intelligence (AI) and brain-computer interfaces (BCIs) will define the future of AAC.
> 2. resist disability being framed medically, as a problem to be solved; yet we acknowledge both the pleasures and pains of being disabled.
> 3. declare that people who use AAC—as cyborgs of necessity rather than choice—should have choice and ownership of our technologies.
> 4. challenge notions of independence as the necessary end goal for disabled bodies and consider interdependence as a human right.
> 5. imagine alternative futures in which all people who use AAC are accepted and embraced for our communication and self-expression.
>
> *(Sellwood et al., 2024)*

Higher value is often placed on powered communication aids, and specifically new and emerging technologies, with comparatively less value being given to paper and partner-based AAC strategies. This message is inequitable considering that newer technologies are often high-cost and therefore inaccessible to many. This over-positive framing of technologies as a solution to communication disability has been termed "technoableism". Placing such value on technology as being capable of "fixing" or "solving" disability sits within the medical model. Instead, practitioners should listen to the views of AAC users regarding what works and what they want, giving them the same authority which is provided to other disabled communities (Robinson, 2018; Sellwood et al., 2024; Shew, 2023).

Value is also placed on speech output over other communication modalities. A more inclusive society is one where all ways of communicating are seen as equally valuable and celebrated. Those working with AAC users might support them to develop a sense of pride about their identity through openly discussing communication differences and difficulties, giving AAC users the language they need to talk about themselves and including them in conversations about equity, diversity and belonging (Bogart, Lund and Rottenstein, 2018).

In order to develop the understanding and acceptance of diverse communication styles, practitioners might reflect on the following questions:

- To what extent do I value speech over other ways of communicating?
- To what extent do the developmental norms of White, middle-class, speaking children influence my practice (i.e. aiming to achieve perceived "normal" ways of communicating)?
- Am I providing opportunities for AAC users to discuss their identity and communication style?
- Am I providing AAC users with the language they need to talk about themselves to others?

Promoted

The lives of disabled people, including those with communication differences and difficulties, are impacted by politics, societal structures and institutional practices. Stigma is used as a "material, structural force, and a form of power" (Niedbalski, 2023).

Being able to communicate through any language or modality is a human right and in turn allows the fulfilment of other human rights, such as access to employment and education. The world has an aging population and an increasing prevalence of disease and chronic conditions which will likely result in the need for AAC. Despite this, access to assistive technology and AAC services is limited for many, especially those in low- and middle-income countries. It is likely that the prevalence of communication disabilities is underestimated and not fully understood, perhaps because communication differences and difficulties are an invisible disability. Their dynamic nature (changing throughout the day and/or a lifetime) can mean that there are further overlooked by society (Harniss et al., 2015).

Views of disability vary within society, creating a shifting hierarchy of disabilities where communication differences and difficulties are given different levels of importance and stigma. Communication differences and difficulties are more likely to be treated negatively within society compared to other disabilities, creating further marginalisation (Harniss et al., 2015; McLeod and McLeod, 2023). Beyond this still, in a society which values higher intelligence, individuals with communication difficulties and differences that also have a Learning Disability will likely be further marginalised and excluded from accessing AAC (Broomfield, 2023; Harris et al., 2023).

Not only are people with communication differences and difficulties excluded within society in general, they may also be excluded from spaces designed for them, such as disability support groups and activism spaces. Armineh Soorenian writes about the challenges she faces accessing such spaces which are "masculine, middle-class and white" (2023, p. 440) and where her dysarthria meant that she was often misunderstood or ignored and it was presumed she didn't understand. Her attempts to take part in disability activism were met with frequent barriers which damaged her self-esteem. Those with communication differences and difficulties might often be perceived as not being able to understand and their views will go unheard (Soorenian, 2023).

Care pathways and funding streams vary around the world. In the UK, Specialised AAC Services provide powered AAC solutions to those who meet a set of criteria. For those who do not, access to AAC is variable and dependent on geographical area. AAC will often be funded through charities or by families themselves. While some might achieve the AAC equipment they need, there will be limited access to practitioners to support the use of the equipment, both in terms of advice and guidance and ongoing maintenance, repair and replacement. So, while access to funding might be seen to be positive, lack of access to inclusive policies and pathways will continue to exclude those with communication differences and difficulties, maintain barriers and limit their participation (Harniss et al., 2015; Ward, 2023).

BOX 9.3 DAVID DESCRIBES HIS EXPERIENCE OF DISABILITY

"For me, being unable to communicate is far more frustrating than being unable to walk but I don't think that is understood by wider society, including those in power."

David Williams, AAC user

One reason for the underfunding of AAC services is the level of awareness that AAC and its potential benefits. This includes both those who might directly support AAC users and those that fund AAC services (Broomfield, 2023). Lack of research has also been linked to the inequity of AAC policy and practice; often we aren't able to confidently say what works and what doesn't. This makes it challenging to then write and enforce policy around AAC assessment and intervention (Baxter et al., 2012; Ward, 2023; Webb et al., 2019).

There is usually an imbalance of power between practitioners and AAC users, where practitioners are seen as the experts and gatekeepers of services and equipment. Those who work with AAC users must reflect on this and attempt to minimise this power imbalance through involving AAC users and their families in decision making. Practitioners will also often feel powerless, as their ways of working are governed by the policies and practices of the systems they work within. The systemic ideologies can make change feel daunting and perhaps impossible at times. Practitioners might attempt to change practice but find they are met with resistance, both from individuals and institutions. Brea-Spahn and Bauler (2023) encourage practitioners to take a "critical inquiry stance", which begins with naming what is happening in current practice. This practice must then be disrupted by challenging the evidence for and against it. Reflection and action then follow, through conversations, education and resistance to current ways of being. Finally, these new perspectives must be viewed within the context of marginalised communities as practice is reframed.

In order to implement a critical enquiry stance, practitioners might ask themselves the following reflective questions:

- What evidence do I have for the way I am doing things now (for and against)?
- Do my beliefs align with my actions? If not, what are the barriers?
- How comfortable am I challenging and changing my own practice?
- How comfortable am I in challenging the practice of others?
- How can I and do I use my privilege as a perceived expert to influence positive change for AAC users?
- What am I doing to increase awareness of AAC (within my team, at a strategic level, and publicly)?
- To what extent does my own discomfort limit the extent which I discuss AAC with others (e.g., assuming people won't understand, not wanting to explain terminology, assuming lack of interest)?
- What am I doing to highlight the societal and institutional barriers faced by AAC users?

Summary

AAC users face stigma which is perpetuated and enforced through societal structures, policy and practice. Stigma and isolation have been linked to low self-esteem. Like other marginalised groups, disabled people might develop a sense pride through joining together with others like themselves, which has been shown to increase self-esteem and develop a sense of belonging. Practitioners need to be aware on how intersectionality impacts AAC users and educate themselves about the culture of those they work with so that they can better understand how this may impact the way a person engages with AAC support.

AAC interventions are dominated by White, Western, middle-class ideologies of what is normal and are rooted in the medical model, placing higher value on speech compared to other modalities. Atypical communication styles may often be seen as something to fix or change in order to enable individuals to participate in society which favours a standard way of communicating.

Practitioners are encouraged to challenge their beliefs and implicit bias in order to promote AAC acceptance. Policies and practices that are harmful to some people, especially those within marginalised groups, may be linked to lack of awareness about AAC by those in power who have the ability to influence. Practitioners must engage in self-reflection and consider how they might use their own power to promote awareness of AAC, along with acceptance and pride in diverse communication styles.

References

Baxter, S., Enderby, P., Evans, P. and Judge, S. (2012). Interventions using high-technology communication devices: A state of the art review. *Folia Phoniatrica et Logopaedica*, 64(3), 137-144. https://doi.org/10.1159/000338250.

Beverly Vicker, M.S., CCC-SLP. (nd). Communicative functions or purposes of communication. www.iidc.indiana.edu/irca/articles/communicative-functions-or-purposes-of-communication.html.

Bogart, K. (2017, October). Disability pride: Why disability is not a bad thing. *Exceptional Parent Magazine*, 32-33.

Bogart, K. R., Lund, E. M. and Rottenstein, A. (2018). Disability pride protects self-esteem through the rejection-identification model. *Rehabilitation Psychology*, 63(1), 155-159. https://doi.org/10.1037/rep0000166.

Brea-Spahn, M. R. and Bauler, C. V. (2023). Where do you anchor your beliefs? An invitation to interrogate dominant ideologies of language and languaging in speech-language pathology. *Language, Speech, and Hearing Services in Schools*, 54(3), 675-687. https://doi.org/10.1044/2023_LSHSS-22-00135.

Broomfield, K. (2023). Access to Electronic Assistive Technologies: Exploring local services and pathways to access technology for health and care in South Yorkshire. NHS South Yorkshire Integrated Care Board. https://assistivetech.barnsleyhospital.nhs.uk/wp-content/uploads/2023/11/Final_report_EAT-SYICB_Aug2023.pdf.

Chapman, R. (2023). *Empire of Normality: Neurodiversity and Capitalism*. Pluto Press.

Clarke, M. and Kirton, A. (2003). Patterns of interaction between children with physical disabilities using augmentative and alternative communication systems and their peers. *Child Language Teaching and Therapy*, 19(2), 135-151. https://doi.org/10.1191/0265659003ct248oa.

Cushing, I. (2022). Word rich or word poor? Deficit discourses, raciolinguistic ideologies and the resurgence of the "word gap" in England's education policy. *Critical Inquiry in Language Studies*, 1-27. https://doi.org/10.1080/15427587.2022.2102014.

Hall, E. (2010). Spaces of social inclusion and belonging for people with intellectual disabilities. *Journal of Intellectual Disability Research*, 54(s1), 48-57. https://doi.org/10.1111/j.1365-2788.2009.01237.x.

Harniss, M., Samant Raja, D. and Matter, R. (2015). Assistive technology access and service delivery in resource-limited environments: Introduction to a special issue of Disability and Rehabilitation: Assistive Technology. *Disability and Rehabilitation: Assistive Technology*, 10(4), 267-270. https://doi.org/10.3109/17483107.2015.1039607.

Harris, J., Fialka-Feldman, M., Cartier, M. E. and Soldovieri, S. J. (2023). Hierarchies of leadership within disability justice movements. In S. Meyers, M. McCloskey and G. Petri, *The Routledge*

International Handbook of Disability Human Rights Hierarchies (1st ed., pp. 443–459). Routledge. https://doi.org/10.4324/9781003410089-30.

Harvey, S. and Charles, J. J. (2023). The balancing act. In S. Meyers, M. McCloskey and G. Petri, *The Routledge International Handbook of Disability Human Rights Hierarchies* (1st ed., pp. 88–99). Routledge. https://doi.org/10.4324/9781003410089-8.

Communication Matters Conference, Leeds University of Leeds, United Kingdom.

Huer, Mary Blake. (2000). Examining perceptions of graphic symbols across cultures: Preliminary study of the impact of culture/ethnicity. *AAC Augmentative and Alternative Communication*, 16, 180–185.

Joncour, N. (2004). Fighting for the rights of the non-speaking: Typing words to be heard. In S. Meyers, M. McCloskey and G. Petri (eds) *The Routledge International Handbook of Disability Human Rights Hierarchies*. Routledge.

Kewanian, A., Creely, E. and Southcott, J. (2024). Fierce parenting: An autoethnographic study of disability, inclusion, and "othering". *International Journal of Qualitative Studies in Education*, 37(6), 1736–1751. https://doi.org/10.1080/09518398.2023.2203118.

Martin, D., Small, K. and Stevens, R. (2017) *The Pragmatics Profile for People Who Use AAC*, 2nd Edition, Ace Centre.

McLeod, S. and McLeod, J. (2023). Communication rights moderated through hierarchies of disability and childhood. In S. Meyers, M. McCloskey and G. Petri, *The Routledge International Handbook of Disability Human Rights Hierarchies* (1st ed., pp. 362–381). Routledge. https://doi.org/10.4324/9781003410089-24.

Nair, V. K., Farah, W. and Cushing, I. (2023). A critical analysis of standardized testing in speech and language therapy. *Language, Speech, and Hearing Services in Schools*, 54(3), 781–793. https://doi.org/10.1044/2023_LSHSS-22-00141.

Niedbalski, J. (2023). (Extra)ordinary parenting: Parents of children with disabilities in the context of disability stigma and pride. *Journal of Intellectual Disabilities*, 27(3), 648–670. https://doi.org/10.1177/17446295221100037.

Omino, M., Nagesh, S. (2023). Rooted in rights. In S. Meyers, M. McCloskey and G. Petri, *The Routledge International Handbook of Disability Human Rights Hierarchies* (1st ed., pp. 553–571). Routledge.

Pennington, L. and Mcconachie, H. (1999). Mother-child interaction revisited: Communication with non-speaking physically disabled children. *International Journal of Language & Communication Disorders*, 34(4), 391–416. https://doi.org/10.1080/136828299247351.

Pope, L., Light, J. and Franklin, A. (2022). Black children with developmental disabilities receive less augmentative and alternative communication intervention than their White peers: Preliminary evidence of racial disparities from a secondary data analysis. *American Journal of Speech-Language Pathology*, 31(5), 2159–2174. https://doi.org/10.1044/2022_AJSLP-22-00079.

Robinson, H. (2018, March). AAC technology: What's in a name? *Royal College of Speech and Language Therapist's Bulletin*, 11.

Robinson, H. (2023, December 9). *The Positive AAC Framework* [Poster presentation].

Scorgie, K. (with Forlin, C.). (2019). *Promoting Social Inclusion: Co-Creating Environments That Foster Equity and Belonging*. Emerald Publishing Limited.

Sellwood, D., McLeod, L., Williams, K., Brown, K. and Pullin, G. (2024). Imagining alternative futures with augmentative and alternative communication: A manifesto. *Medical Humanities*, medhum-2024-013022. https://doi.org/10.1136/medhum-2024-013022.

Shew, A. (2023). *Against Technoableism: Rethinking Who Needs Improvement (a Norton Short)* (1st ed.). W. W. Norton & Company, Incorporated.

Soorenian, A. (2023). Excluded from the disability rights debate. In S. Meyers, M. McCloskey and G. Petri, *The Routledge International Handbook of Disability Human Rights Hierarchies* (1st ed., pp. 437–442). Routledge. https://doi.org/10.4324/9781003410089-29.

The Keycomm Team. (2011). *The Codes Framework*.

Ward, J. (2023). Disability and displacement. In S. Meyers, M. McCloskey and G. Petri, *The Routledge International Handbook of Disability Human Rights Hierarchies* (1st ed., pp. 301–317). Routledge. https://doi.org/10.4324/9781003410089-20.

Webb, E. J. D., Lynch, Y., Meads, D., Judge, S., Randall, N., Goldbart, J., Meredith, S., Moulam, L., Hess, S. and Murray, J. (2019). Finding the best fit: Examining the decision-making of augmentative and alternative communication professionals in the UK using a discrete choice experiment. *BMJ Open*, 9(11), e030274. https://doi.org/10.1136/bmjopen-2019-030274.

Yu, B., Epstein, L. and Tisi, V. (2021). A DisCrit-informed critique of the difference vs. disorder approach in speech-language pathology. In R. Horton (ed.), *Advances in Linguistics and Communication Studies* (pp. 105–128). IGI Global. https://doi.org/10.4018/978-1-7998-7134-7.ch006.

Appendices

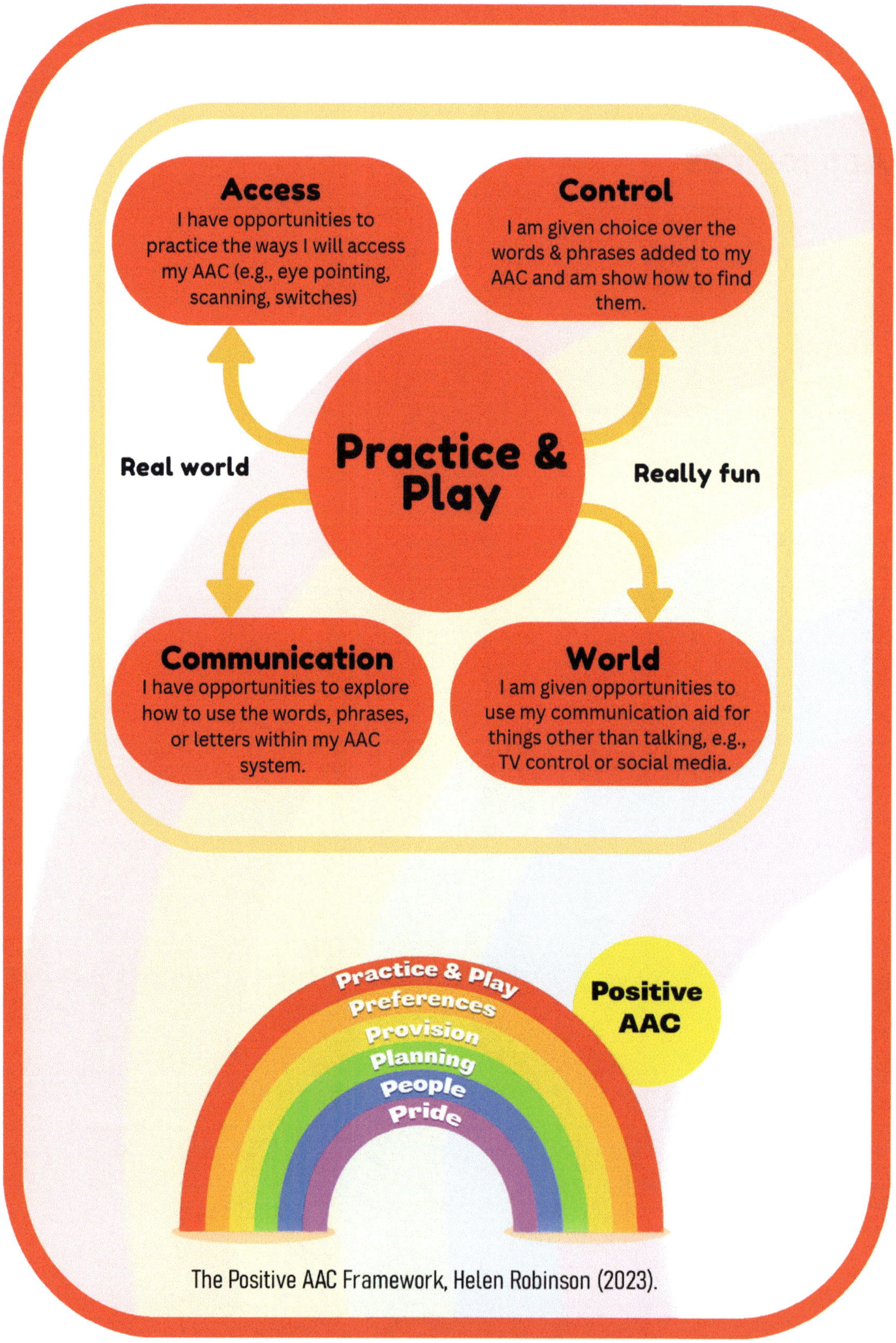
Access
I have opportunities to practice the ways I will access my AAC (e.g., eye pointing, scanning, switches)
Control
I am given choice over the words & phrases added to my AAC and am show how to find them.
Real world
Practice & Play
Really fun
Communication
I have opportunities to explore how to use the words, phrases, or letters within my AAC system.
World
I am given opportunities to use my communication aid for things other than talking, e.g., TV control or social media.
Practice & Play
Preferences
Provision
Planning
People
Pride
Positive AAC
The Positive AAC Framework, Helen Robinson (2023).

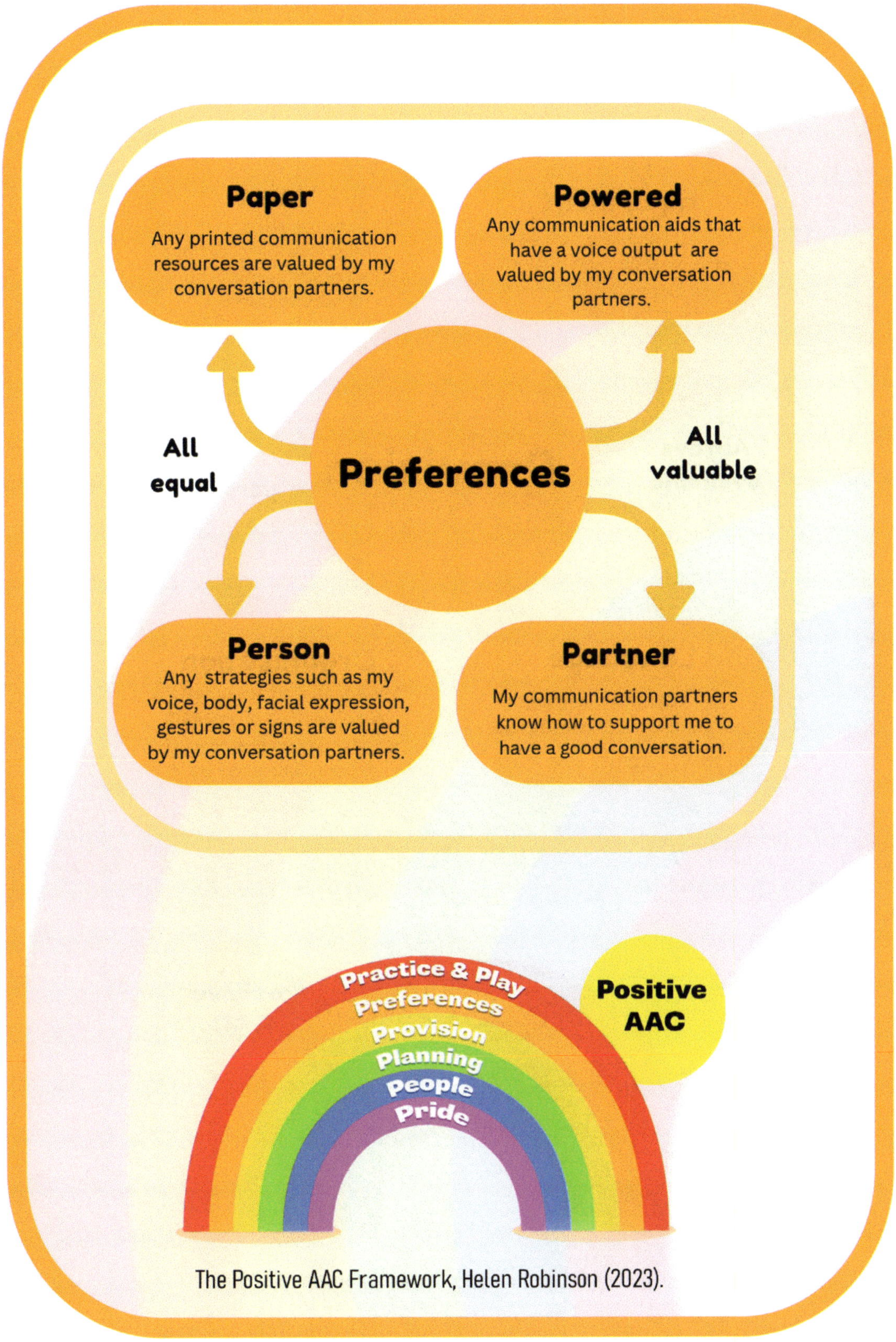

The Positive AAC Framework, Helen Robinson (2023).

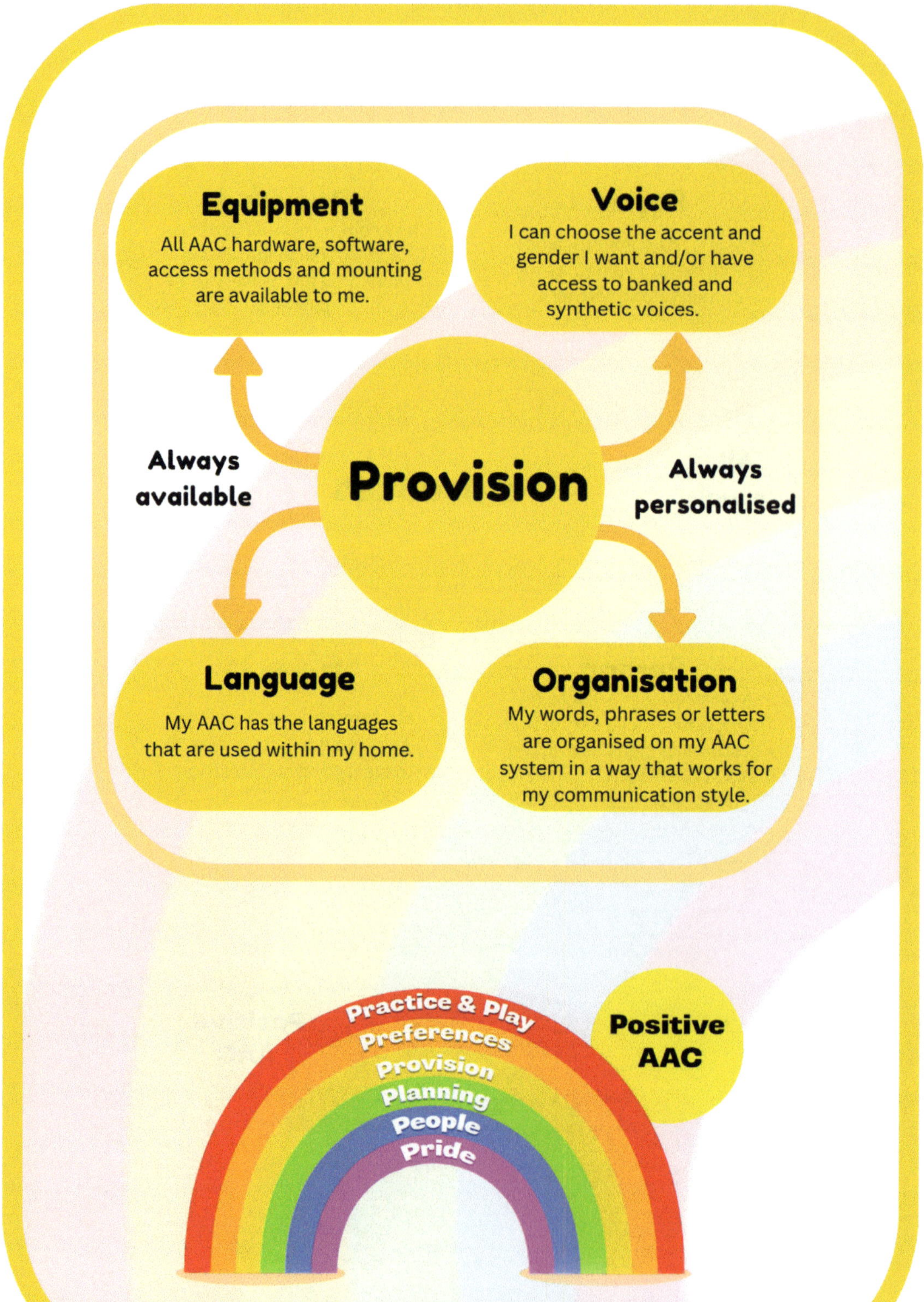

The Positive AAC Framework, Helen Robinson (2023).

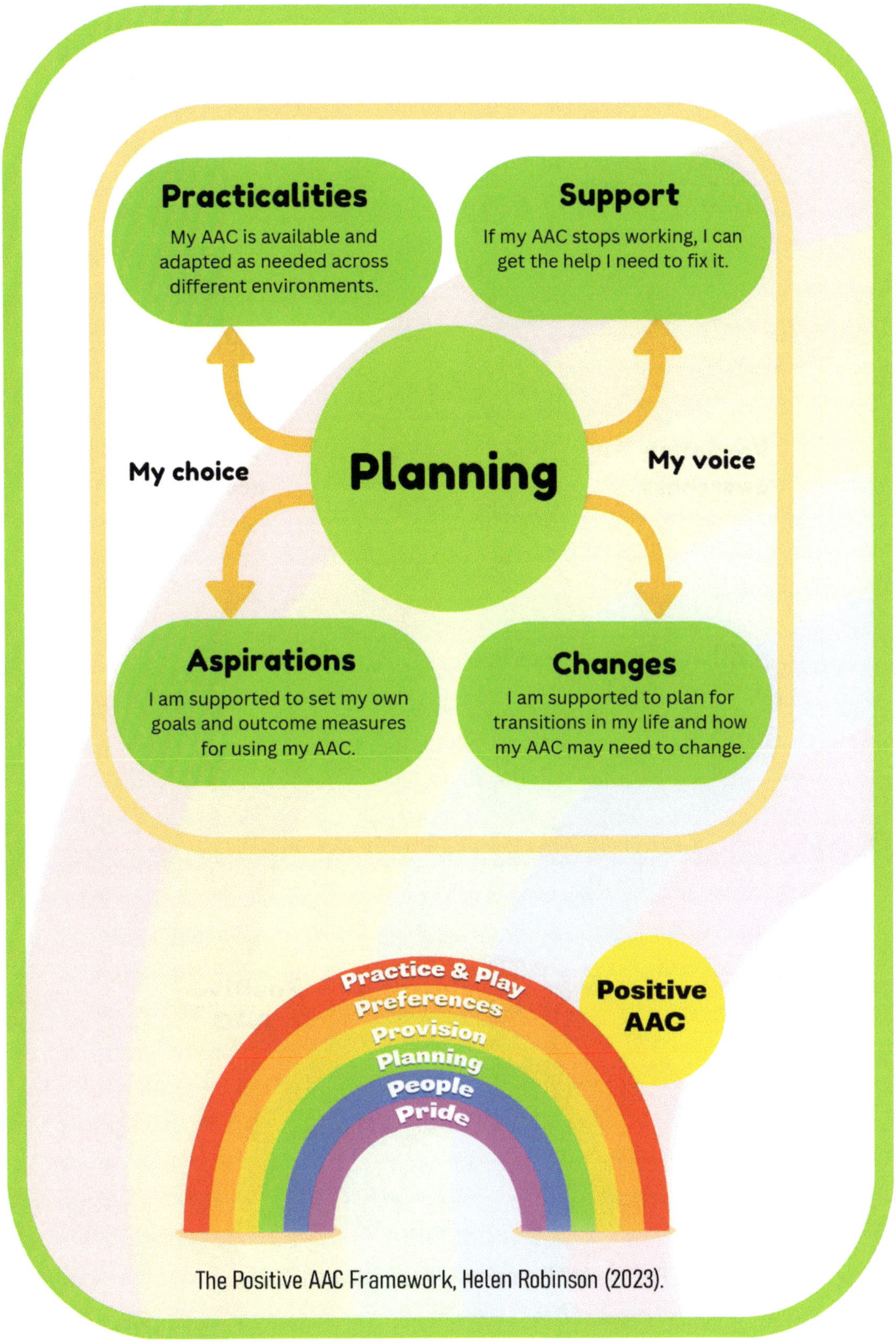

The Positive AAC Framework, Helen Robinson (2023).

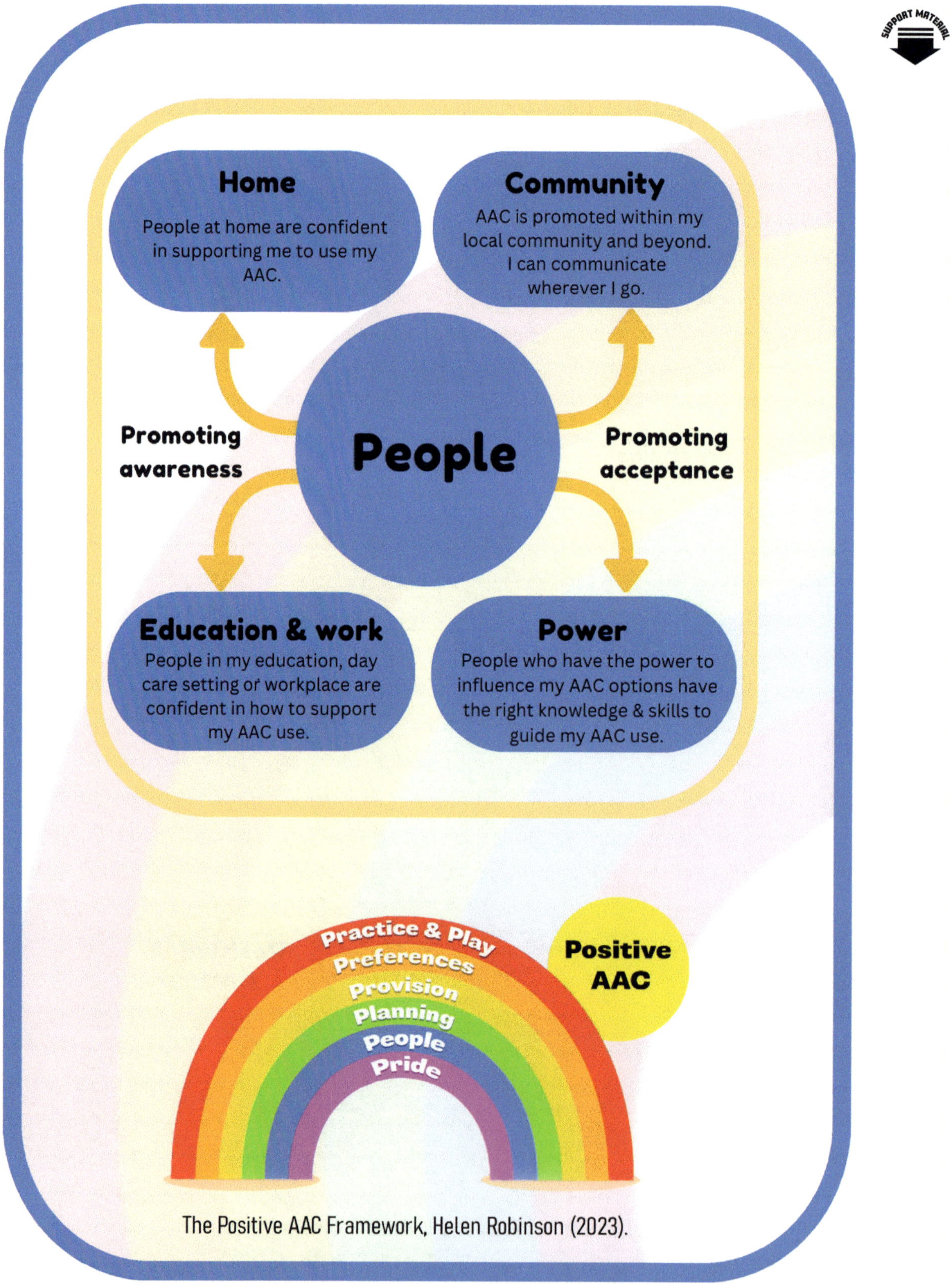

The Positive AAC Framework, Helen Robinson (2023).

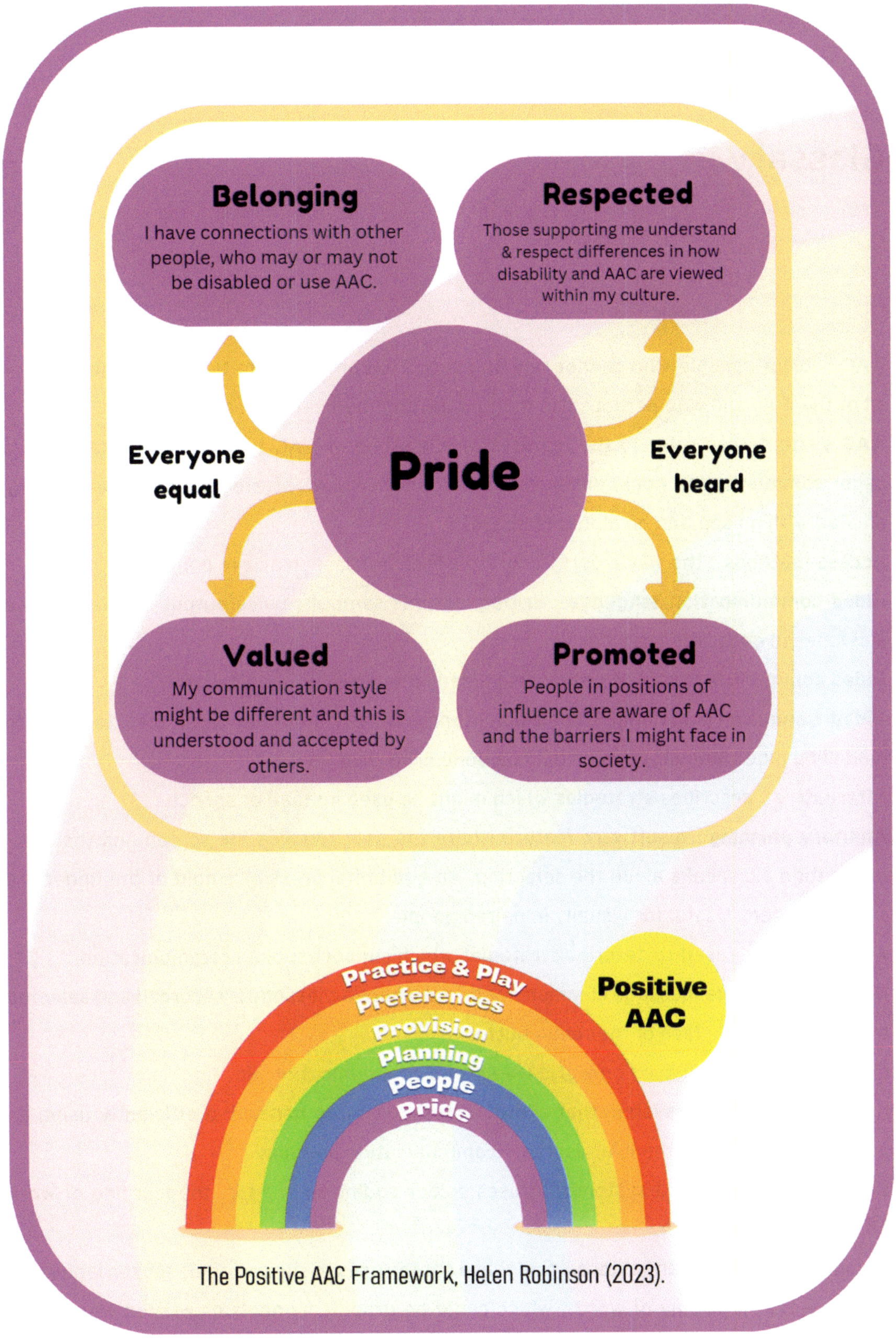

The Positive AAC Framework, Helen Robinson (2023).

Glossary

AAC user(s) people who cannot rely on speech to communicate their message some or all of the time and who perhaps use multimodal communication in a unique way.

AAC system can refer to the features of one mode of AAC that a person uses (e.g., a paper communication book) or a collection of all their AAC strategies (e.g., eye pointing, an iPad with an app and an alphabet board).

Access methods the way a person controls their AAC, such as eye pointing or touch.

Aided communication/language writing, graphic symbols, voice output communication aids/speech generating devices.

Aided communicators people who use aided language/communication.

Aided Language Modelling/Stimulation Approach an umbrella term used to refer to modelling aided language, which may be done is several ways.

Alternative describes strategies which might be used instead of speech.

Auditory phishing a software feature where the user touches the screen and the communication aid speaks aloud the selection. An additional press or a hold of the finger will select the item. Useful for visually impaired people.

Augmentative used to describe strategies which support spoken communication.

Big Mack a single message communication aid where a message is recorded and selected by pressing the surface of the round button.

Cells the items displayed on a grid layout of a communication aid.

Coding/encoding a system that allows a message to be generated efficiently using an agreed code between the AAC user and communication partner.

Colourful semantics a system that uses colour coding to support the learning of word order.

Communication aid any external tool that a person uses to support their spoken language.

Core boards a display of words, which could be graphic symbols or written words that represent high frequency words chosen from core word lists.

Core vocabulary words/concepts which occur most frequently in a language.

Dedicated device a tablet or computer which is designed specifically to be used as a communication aid.

Delayed echolalia the repetition of language after it has been heard, not in the moment.

Device a term often used to refer to voice output communication aids.

Dynamic displays vocabulary packages where selecting an item navigates the user to a different page.

Echolalia the repetition of language either in the moment or at a later point.

Electromyography (EMG) the measurement of electrical signals produced by muscles which can be used to control a switch for access to technology.

Environmental controls an umbrella terms used for assistive technology which allows people to access mainstream technology such as televisions, mobile phones or door intercoms which they would otherwise not be able to control.

Expert model the idea that professionals know better than the person with lived experience and should carry the power to make decisions about what's best for the person.

Facilitated communication a communication partner supports the person to communicate by providing physical support, such as holding their elbow.

Fitzgerald Key the colour coding of words and/or graphic symbols according to word groups.

Fringe vocabulary words and phrases related to topics and activities, often nouns, and highly personal to the individual.

Graphic symbols pictures or icons that represent concepts.

Hardware the physical equipment containing the language, such as the communication book, E-tran frame, or tablet computer.

Head mouse a camera either integrated into the computer screen, or a peripheral device, tracks head movements and converts this to the movement of a mouse cursor.

Identity-first language a way to describe someone using a label first, e.g., AAC user, autistic person.

Motor planning theory the idea that we learn patterns to remember where items are located, e.g., the numeric code to unlock a door or a phone, or touch typing on a keyboard.

Mounting options the ways in which a communication aid can be fixed to a mount, which might be free standing on a floor or table, or attached to a wheelchair.

Multi-meaning symbols a graphic symbol which changes meaning when combined with another.

Multimodal (communicator) the use of a range of strategies to communicate, e.g., speech, writing and a communication aid.

Organisational method the way in which these graphic symbols, photographs, letters or written words are arranged within the vocabulary package.

Paper-based AAC AAC using paper or printed resources e.g. a paper symbol board or an E-tran frame.

Partner assisted scanning the communication partner points to or read out items in turn for the AAC user to select.

Patient reported outcome measures (PROMS) a tool that allows service users to measure the impact of the support they receive.

Person first language a way to describe someone beginning with "person with ..." or "person who ..." The diagnostic label comes after, e.g., person with autism.

Powered AAC/Powered communication aids communication aids using a plug or batteries, usually with voice output.

Pragmatic branch starters a phrase which sets the context or pragmatic function of a message, e.g., "I'm asking a question" or "I want something".

Pragmatically organised vocabulary a way of organising language on a communication aid via communicative functions, e.g., asking questions, describing something, telling a story.

Pragmatic Organisation Dynamic Display (PODD©) a commercially available AAC system in either printed form or computer software.

Schematic vocabulary is organised around an event or activity.

Semantic compaction sequences of icons are combined to produce words or phrases based on linguistic rules

Speech generating device communication aids which produce voice which might be recorded or synthesised

Static overlay communication aids/displays AAC systems with just one page that doesn't change.

Switch a peripheral device that allows a user to control an electronic device.

Symbol sets collections of symbols without internal logic, usually where each symbol has a single meaning.

Symbol systems collections of symbols which hold internal logic and can generate new meanings.

Synthetic voice design two or more samples of speech are blended to produce a new voice.

Talking Mats a visual communication framework used to gain the views of AAC users.

Taxonomic in AAC, the term used to describe the organisation of language by categories, e.g., food, animals.

Unaided communication ways of communicating without an external system, e.g., speech, gestures, facial expression.

User Centred Design the views of those who will use the product are actively sought and included in the design process.

Visual scenes a photograph is used either to set the context of the communication, with graphic symbols next to it, or "hot spots" are assigned where the person touches a spot in the photo to elicit a symbol or spoken word/phrase.

Vocabulary package a term used to describe a commercially available language system which can often be edited by the user. It might be used on a communication aid or printed on paper.

Voice banking a person records their speech to turn into a synthetic voice which may later be used on a communication aid.

Voice Input Voice Output communication aids (VIVOCAs) the user speaks a word (which may be unintelligible to a communication partner) and the software translates it into text or synthetic voice output.

Voice Output communication Aids (VOCAs) communication aids which produce recorded or synthesised voice.

Voice repair unclear speech can be recorded and repaired to turn it into a synthetic voice which sounds like the individual.

Index

For Product Safety Concerns and Information please contact our EU representative GPSR@taylorandfrancis.com Taylor & Francis Verlag GmbH, Kaufingerstraße 24, 80331 München, Germany

* 9 7 8 1 0 3 2 5 3 4 8 9 3 *

T - #0033 - 220725 - C284 - 297/210/13 - SB - 9781032534893 - Gloss Lamination